W9-AQE-297

Patient Care and Rehabilitation of Communication-Impaired Adults

PATIENT CARE AND REHABILITATION OF COMMUNICATION-IMPAIRED ADULTS

By

RALPH R. LEUTENEGGER, Ph.D.

Department of Speech Pathology and Audiology
University of Wisconsin-Milwaukee
Milwaukee, Wisconsin

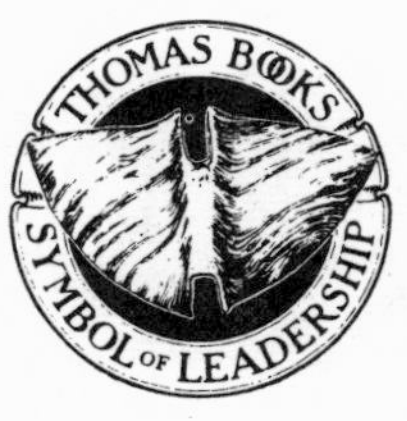

CHARLES C THOMAS • PUBLISHER
Springfield • Illinois • U.S.A.

Published and Distributed Throughout the World by

CHARLES C THOMAS • PUBLISHER
Bannerstone House
301-327 East Lawrence Avenue, Springfield, Illinois, U.S.A.

ISBN 0-398-03473-7

Library of Congress Catalog Card Number: 75-12925

With THOMAS BOOKS *careful attention is given to all details of manufacturing and design. It is the Publisher's desire to present books that are satisfactory as to their physical qualities and artistic possibilities and appropriate for their particular use.* THOMAS BOOKS *will be true to those laws of quality that assure a good name and good will.*

Printed in the United States of America
R-1

Library of Congress Cataloging in Publication Data

Leutenegger, Ralph R
Patient care and rehabilitation of communication-impaired adults.

Bibliography: p.
Includes index.
1. Communicative disorders--Rehabilitation. 2. Aged --Rehabilitation. 3. Speech therapy. I. Title.
[DNLM: 1. Rehabilitation--In old age. 2. Patient care team. 3. Aging. 4. Hearing disorders--Rehabilitation. 5. Speech disorders--Rehabilitation. WT104 L654p]
RC423.L42 362.6′11′9855 75-12925
ISBN 0-398-03473-7

To Jeanette and Fran
and the memory of their two Pauls

PREFACE

THIS book is intended for everyone involved in rehabilitation and in care of the aging. It contains information of value to all of the many professionals, paraprofessionals, and nonprofessionals who come into contact with the patient. The core around which the book revolves is the patient's communication skills and the important roles they play in his total rehabilitation and/or adjustment. The book was written to fill the need expressed by directors of in-service training programs for information appropriate to the staffs in their hospitals, nursing homes, or homes for the aged.

The attending nurse, aides of all types, the physical therapist, the occupational therapist, the psychologist, the rehabilitation counselor, the social worker, the case's family, his clergyman, his physician — these and all others associated in any way with rehabilitation efforts — are frequently baffled as a result of their unawareness of the extent and nature of a patient's communication disruptions. Frequently a patient's seeming belligerence or inattention is ascribed to a nasty disposition rather than recognized as part of his total symptom complex. Thorough assessment of communication skills can play a major role in diagnostic, prognostic, and therapeutic processes.

Why do some rehabilitation (and some maintenance) efforts succeed better than others? This book makes the modest assertion that success might partially be a function of the skills of the staff speech pathologist. It posits the speech pathologist as a necessary team member — one skilled both in direct services to the case, and in an indirect consultative role to all team members including the case and his family. (Similarly the speech pathologist expects to gain from the consultative efforts of every other member of a given case's rehabilitation team, professional members and nonprofessionals alike).

This book was written as a result of the author's growing concern over the widely diverse levels of understanding, by health and health-related workers, of various types of adult communication impairment. The efficient functioning of chronically ill or aged persons is directly related to the degree of understanding that all of the involved health-related workers have of communication breakdowns. This book is intended to help not only the patients, but also to assist those entrusted with their care to greater personal job satisfactions arising from more effective interaction with their patients. While the book is geared to adult cases, the basic concepts of interprofessional relationships and understanding are as pertinent to individuals serving children with specialized communication needs as to those working primarily with adults.

While this book gives detailed information on relating with adults who evince varying degrees of communication breakdown, it does not purport to train all of its readers to be speech and hearing clinicians. Nor does it suggest that this is desirable, much less feasible. The author merely infers that all who come into contact with rehabilitation cases can themselves function more effectively if their training includes meaningful insights into the complex interrelationship that exists between a patient's communication disabilities and health maintenance and rehabilitation practices. For example, the nurse who is apprised of her patient's inability to comprehend long spoken sentences will restrict her questions and comments to simple, commonly-used words and brief phrases, or will communicate in writing — if that communication channel is less affected. The physical therapist will be alerted to more accurately ascertain whether the patient truly cannot perform a given task, or whether he fails to understand the task being required in his muscle reeducation program. The occupational therapist, aware of a homonymous hemianopsia, will work with the speech pathologist on improving the various movement skills subserving reading retraining.

Although the primary focus of this book is on aspects of speech and hearing, it should prove as valuable to other professionals as to speech pathologists. A major goal was to present ideas as simply as possible without the camouflage of unnecessary terminology. The author has struggled too long with other professions' terminology to create knowingly similar problems for others. For example, "BK" invokes in the minds of many speech pathologists reference to an electronic instrumentation company. It took me some time to realize that "BK therapy" referred to procedures "below the knee" rather than therapy utilizing a piece of BK equipment. In conversation recently, the author was perplexed by a public health nurse's obvious difficulty in grasping the meaning of "PICA scores." It turned out that she was well aware of "pica" as a craving for unnatural articles of food, but had not previously known of the aphasia diagnostic test, the Porch Index of Communicative Ability, commonly referred to as the "PICA." An uproariously funny situation occurred when a physician acquaintance finally understood why the hospital's speech pathologist was so delighted in successfully getting his case to produce an acceptable /r/ sound *in isolation*. The author has assiduously attempted, wherever clarity permitted, to minimize the use of professional jargon specific to the speech and hearing profession.

This book extracts materials from the vast literature available on attempts of the ill and aging to cope better within their own home, community rehabilitation center, hospital, nursing home, or residential home for the aged. It particularly singles out for detailed treatment the hard-of-hearing, the poststroke case (both right and left hemiplegics), the multiple sclerotic, the laryngectomee, and individuals diagnosed to have Parkinson's disease.

It is hoped that in some small way this book may help to break down some of the unnecessary professional defenses which are inimical to the best patterns of patient care. For example, I have found physical and occupational therapists who work diligently with the members of a hemiplegic's family teaching them transfer activities, yet who question the speech pathologist's need to have similar skills. I know speech pathologists who give intensive training in language restitution techniques to the mate of an aphasic, but who question giving similar help to nurses, occupational therapists, etc. It is recognized that each profession concentrates in depth upon a given aspect of the patient's well-being. However, it seems to me that an overly rigid interpretation of one's professional boundaries hinders cooperation with other professionals who likewise seek ethically to bring about patient improvement within their own sphere of competency. To assist in achieving better mutual understanding, the book includes a chapter on the roles, training, and certification or licensure procedures required for the various specialists most crucially involved in related direct patient care practices.

At the risk of appearing to claim for speech and hearing too large a role in patient care, I must emphasize the all-pervasive consequences of communication breakdowns to daily living, and particularly to rehabilitation and maintenance concerns. Recognition is given, in the total health care process, to the centrality of the patient *as a communicator*.

Over an extended period of time the author has studied the elements of interprofessional cooperation and possible causes of *team* inadequacies. The recent burgeoning of colleges and schools of health-related professions is one visible cultural manifestation of attempts to cope with some of the concerns felt by the author, many of which he has hoped to alleviate or minimize through the writing of this book. The author will be indeed grateful for whatever small role it can perform in enabling us to understand each other better (our roles, our competencies, our ethical concerns and restrictions, etc.) and to ply our professional skills with the greatest possible gain to our mutual cases and to each other.

ACKNOWLEDGMENTS

My primary indebtedness for whatever discernment this book may reveal is to the clinical cases and their families whom I have been privileged to see professionally over a period of a quarter of a century. The challenge of the problems faced by these individuals and the relative paucity and inaccessibility of help from the clinical literature spurred me on in my quest for additional solutions.

The quest led to offering an experimental seminar in 1967 which dealt with the communication problems of the chronically ill and the aged, and probed ways in which needs of these individuals might be met. Student reaction was so favorable that a new graduate level course was created.

I am indebted to the students who for the subsequent five years enrolled in "The Speech Pathologist's Role with the Chronically Ill and Aged," and to the many people who as guest lecturers participated in the laudatory process of extending our mutual horizons.

These people, along with others who reacted to early drafts of selected chapters of this book, represent the professions of dentistry, community health education, deaf education, hospital administration, medical school administration, medicine, the ministry, nursing, nursing home administration, occupational therapy, physical therapy, rehabilitation counseling, social work, and speech pathology and audiology. For their stimulation and insights, my deep gratitude is extended to Thelma Adkeson, Agatha Armstrong, Sue Benner, Victor Bolle, Laura Braunel, Bernice Brynelson, June Carr, Richard Cooperrider, Dennis Cult, Andrew Cyrus, Roger Dahlberg, Thomas Domato, William T.

Eggers, Mary Finn, Richard Flynn, Mary Kay Gumper Galindo, Jaunita Gillgren, Sally Godozi, June Grommes, Julia Haese, George Handy, Janet Harvey, Emma Heller, Philip Hoyer, Carmen Ilseman, Edward Jimenez-Pabon, John C. Jorgensen, Eleanor Jorgenson, Marjorie Jothen, Gale Kelly, Lee Knox, Elizabeth A. Krueger, Gerard Kupperman, Max Kurz, Frieda Laubach, Harriet Lazinski, Basilio Lopez, Mary J. Marks, Karen Metzger, Mary Neuman, Colette Oberembt, Fred Phlughoeft, Rev. Rem, Betty Ritchie, Earl Rosen, Timothy Ryan, Dave Schlesinger, Antoinette Scott, Stanley Sehler, Sidney Shindell, Janice Stovall, Ann Trotter, Mary Verfurth, Warren von Ehren, Jordan Weigler, Bonnie Weissenfluh, Edwin Welsh, Betty Westphal, and Arthur Zolecki.

Very special thanks are extended to the following, all of whom at the time of their contributions to my class, were consultants in the Patient Care Practices section of the Wisconsin Division of Health — Agatha Armstrong, Laura Braunel, John C. Jorgensen, Eleanor Jorgenson, Lee Knox, Frieda Laubach, and Janice Stovall. These health consultant pioneers not only passed on the benefit of their classroom teaching skills, but several of them, Janice Stovall in particular, enabled my students to observe them as they applied their consultant skills in nursing homes and homes for the aged. We gained immeasurably from your instruction.

It is with pleasure and appreciation that I recognize the stimulation received from the many people associated with the seminar "Speech Pathology and Audiology Services Under Medicare and Medicaid" held at the Catholic University of America in Washington D.C., May 16 through 18, 1969, and with the ASHA-PHS Region V Seminar of the same name, held in Milwaukee, Wisconsin, May 15 through 17, 1970.

In a similar vein, I am grateful to all who participated in the Indiana Regional Medical Program's short Course "Perspectives on a Rehabilitation Theme: Interdisciplinary Function in Patient Care," held in Nashville, Indiana, September 24 through 26, 1970.

In addition, I wish to thank the innumerable staff members of various hospitals and nursing homes in southeastern Wisconsin who have so graciously and generously cooperated in helping to educate me and my students.

For insights uniquely ralated to the contents of this book I am obligated to my long-time friend Dr. McKenzie Buck, his wife Betty, and their children Bill and Judy. My knowledge of this family's interactions before, during, and after Dr. Buck's series of strokes has been a constant inspiration in my attempts to be of help and assurance to otehr families facing similar problems.

As is frequently the case with acknowledgments, my final expression of indebtedness is the most heartfelt and meaningful. I wish to thank the remarkable woman who married me during student days — Beth Louise Wilimek Leutenegger — and who carried the brunt of the load of raising five children while her husband besieged libraries, hospitals, nursing homes, patients, and all manner of professionals in an attempt to improve patient care practices. I sincerely trust that whatever gains may accrue from this book to adults with communication problems, that they somehow compensate for the many hours that this project has stolen from my wife and children.

R.R.L.

CONTENTS

Patient Care and Rehabilitation of Communication-Impaired Adults

Chapter 1

CHANGES IN AGING

As we look about us at friends and at strangers, we cannot help but notice the side effects of a youth-oriented society. Business executives and top salesmen are crowding the society matrons in the plastic surgeon's offices for face-lifts. Overnight, sparse hair becomes supplanted by thicker thatch in the form of wigs. For the more affluent, hair implants are replacing departing "first crops." The advent of contact lenses enabled many people to return from the near blindness their vanity committed them to because of an aversion to wearing glasses. Similarly, hearing aids have been rejected as a threat to the individual's ego image.

As a nation we tend to be reluctant to admit normal physical and physiological decline. Glasses and hearing aids emphasize the "losing" aspects of aging. Our glorification of youth causes definite hang-ups about age. Despite rejection or battling, old age will catch up with most of us — ecology, hypertension, cigarettes, alcohol, wars, and the highways willing.

The majority of the professionals reading this book, while they are probably victims of the youth-cult themselves, demand candor on the part of their clients, cases, or patients, and the families of those they serve. This book will attempt to reflect that candor in briefly listing some of the major changes that occur to the individual with the passing years. Any given communication impairment needs to be evaluated in relationship to such changes.

It is interesting to note that the true primary cause of aging remains unknown. Indeed, there is little in the professional literature to help the medical practitioner compare his older patients with ranges of normal function appropriate to given ages. Information on such physical profiles of aging is relatively scant. This makes it exceedingly difficult to assess where physiology ends and pathology begins. How should people be expected to react within the restrictions of their age?

It is true that "an aged human being usually can be recognized by the appearance of his skin and hair, his speed of movement, his gait, his posture and the degree of loss of his vigor and vitality. Nevertheless, these are only the reflection of a number of inner changes in structure, in chemical make-up, and in functional effectiveness of various organs of the body and their component parts" (U.S. Dept. of HEW, 1970).

Organic degeneration brings about fatigability — stairs become harder to climb, streets become more dangerous to cross, parcels become heavier to carry. Artificial assistance (i.e. false teeth, spectacles, hearing aids, walking-sticks) become necessary to carry out one's natural functions. While there are changes in an individual's appearance which enable us to estimate his age within a few years, there is a wide variation in how systems change.

Let us begin by looking at the *skin and subcutaneous tissues.* With increasing age the skin becomes dry and flabby, losing its elasticity. It begins to wrinkle, becoming parchment-like. Increased pigmentation is discernable in the appearance of brown spots. The upper lip becomes thinner. Earlobes increase in size. The eyelids thicken, and hollows develop beneath the eyes. Hair becomes dry and brittle. It greys, whitens, and drops out. It grows sparse, particularly on the head. However, it also appears in new places, such as on the chins of old women. Teeth decay and drop out. It is estimated that two thirds of the population are endentulous (toothless) by the age of 75. This loss of teeth brings about a shortening of the lower part of the face — the chin comes nearer to the nose. Finger-and toenails become harder, thicker, and ridged.

Extensive changes are also detected in the *skeletal system.* With compression of the spinal discs, the vertebrae come closer together. Our posture is affected by bowing of the spine, decrease in chest measurements, and narrowing of the shoulders. At the same time, the pelvis becomes broader. Muscular strength declines. Muscular atrophy and sclerosis of the joints (becoming stiff and creaky) lead to difficulties in moving. The person begins to shuffle and totter. Chronic arthritis impairs the limbs, back, and trunk. This common disease is a painful disorder which affects joints and their supporting muscles, cartilages, and connective tissue. There is a shrinking of the gums, which results in ill-fitting teeth. The auditory canal shrinks, rendering earmolds less efficient.

Probably the most important system in aging is the *cardiovascular system*. The heart, which helps to distribute nutrients and remove wastes, becomes smaller and deteriorates in its functioning. Heart valves and arteries lose their elasticity. There is a decrease in the amount of blood pumped. To counterbalance this decrease, the person reduces his activity. The circulatory system is seriously affected by the development of arteriosclerosis. Cerebral circulation is diminished; the brain's consumption of oxygen diminishes. This reduction in oxygen content brings about a slowing-down of the conceptual processes, a reduction in immediate memory and in retention, irregularity in simple mental operations, and very strong emotional reactions such as euphoria or depression. The veins lose their elasticity. Blood pressure rises.

The *respiratory system* also undergoes change. There is a loss of elasticity in the lungs, causing them to hold less air. With a decrease in respiratory capacity, there is a decrease in oxygen consumption. Breathing becomes difficult. The thoracic cage becomes more rigid because of muscular atrophy and sclerosis of the joints. In addition to muscle atrophy in the rib cage, similar atrophy develops in the larynx, the pharynx, and the trachea.

The *gastrointestinal tract* loses muscle tone, leading to constipation. The digestive system is indirectly affected by the shrinking of the mandible and maxilla, leading to loss of teeth. The salivary glands become less active, resulting in dryness in the mouth. Degeneration in the kidneys, liver, and digestive glands results in reduced filtering.

Changes in both male and female are evident in the *reproductive system and endocrine glands*. There is a diminution in sexual response. It is heartening to note a very few motion picture producers tackling the subject of sex in the aged for purposes other than ridicule — such as in the film, *Harold and Maude** There would probably be far fewer confused and disgusted children, grandchildren, and mates if the following positive approach were more generally known and accepted: "the most important advice that practitioners can give the elderly with reference to sexual relations is that as long as they maintain sexual desire and are able to satisfy this desire, they should not consider this activity in any way abnormal or inappropriate" (U.S. Dept. of HEW, 1969).

The *central nervous system* (brain and spinal cord) also degenerates due to cell disintegration. Reactions become slower as a result of the weakening of sensory input.

The *special senses* of vision and hearing which afford us contact with sound waves and light waves, supply us with less and less environmental stimulation. The sense of vision, since it gives only one half of a sphere for orientation, does not give total security. With the passing years, the power of visual accommodation diminishes. In particular, there is difficulty in adapting to darkness. Presbyopea (farsightedness) is an almost universal phenomenon, rendering glasses a necessity for seeing things which are near. Increasing age brings an increasing incidence of glaucoma (increased pressure within the eyeball), cataract (opacity of the lens, obstructing passage of light waves), and blindness.

Hearing is our chief means of orientation since it puts us in the center of a sphere at all times; it gives information on every vector. It not only gives an assessment of distance, but of proximity as well. Deafness is frequently associated with paranoid behavior patterns. "Decreased hearing sensitivity in elderly persons often causes limitations of social relationships and enjoyment of activities such as church attendance, radio, concerts, television, and social visiting" (U.S. Dept. of HEW, 1969).

We can more readily understand some of the consequences of ear pathologies when we consider the two functions of the ear as an organ. Cochlear problems include disturbances of hearing and

---

**Harold and Maude*, directed by Hall Ashby, produced by Paramount, and starring Ruth Gordon and Bud Cort, was released in December, 1971.

ringing in the ears; vestibular functions include the governing of balance and position in space.

The special senses of touch, taste, and smell all become less sensitive than they were. Light touch on the soles of the feet aids in gravity and balance. With lessened sensitivity comes imperfect balance. Lessened environmental stimulation causes one to live in a less vibrant world. When we consider the statement "the world is as each being perceives it," we can easily understand how drastically life is changed with diminution of the effectiveness of the various senses. Indeed, "behavioral scientists have shown that they can induce irritability, confusion, delusions, and even hallucinations in a matter of a few hours by depriving normal healthy young persons of normal sensory inputs" (Fowler and Fordyce, 1972).

Frequently, impairment in the ability to communicate is viewed as the greatest geriatric burden of all. Diminution of visual and auditory acuity impairs the patient's reception of spoken or written information. Irreversible changes in movement of the tongue, jaw, lips, soft palate, and vocal folds, as well as cerebral deterioration involving language processes, result in the inability to speak as one formerly did.

Impaired ability to verbally express one's needs, emotions, and reactions, and impairment of the ability to understand linguistic symbols, will invariably create problems of social adjustment and control, leading to withdrawal and isolation. Confusion, anxiety, depressions, or euphoria — these are frequent concomitants of the reduction in communication skills.

It would be remiss to view old age solely from the biological standpoint. In order to understand old age, one must also view it as a cultural fact. "The words 'a fine old age,' 'a green old age,' mean that the elderly person has found a physical and mental balance, and not that his physical being, his memory and his possibilities of psychomotor adaptation are those of a young man" (deBeauvoir, 1972).

For professionals who desire to serve effectively the chronically ill and the aged, it is mandatory to understand that "factors hampering learning in old age include: (1) insufficient response time, (2) stress or arousal of anxiety in the learning situation, (3) lack of motivation of the subject, (4) difficulty in discriminating between environmental stimuli, and (5) psycho-motor deficits in responding to such stimuli" (Pincus, 1968).

Aging, necessarily, is a process of adjusting to dependency, to a loss of resources. As indicated in the preceding pages, there is a decline in physical and physiological health (strength diminishes, appearance changes, sex drive diminishes, an awareness of the prospect of death develops). In the social sphere, one must adjust to the loss of family, friends, associates, prestige, social status, respect, and one's job. The socioeconomic sphere subjects the individual to financial insecurity; he becomes the victim of inflation. Emotional changes result from financial factors and the assumption of new roles, or from "disengagement."* Psychological functioning suffers due to memory impairment, reduced resiliency. All of these diminishing resources complicate previously existing deficits, such as overdependency on one's mate or on the family doctor.

Grief and depression become handy reactions to loss of special skills, prestige, legally or socially invested powers, family, friends, etc. While attempting to face the problems of everyday life, helplessness, hopelessness, fear, anger, and failure — real or anticipated — interfere with self-esteem. Such feelings are further complicated by the the individual's personal reactions to his declining organ functions, etc.

Simone deBeauvoir has most eloquently called attention to the plight of our aged by noting that

> If old people show the same desires, the same feelings and the same requirements as the young, the world looks upon them with disgust: in them love and jealousy seem revolting or absurd, sexuality repulsive and violence ludicrous. They are required to be a standing example of all the virtues. Above all they are called upon to display serenity: the world asserts that they possess it, and this assertion allows the world to ignore their unhappiness. The purified image of themselves that

---

*Cumming and Henry define *disengagement* as "an inevitable process in which many of the relationships between a poerson and other members of society are severed, and those remaining are altered in quality" (Elaine Cumming and William E. Henry, *Growing Old — The Process of Disengagement* [New Y9rk, Basic Books, 1961]).

> society offers the aged is that of the white-haired and venerable sage, rich in experience, planning high above the common state of mankind: if they vary from this, then they fall below it. The counterpart of the first image is that of the old fool in his dotage, a laughing-stock for children. In any case, either by their virtue or by their degradation, they stand outside humanity (deBeauvoir, 1972).

Ruth Baumann, in *Public and Private Partnership for Older Americans,* sets forth the priorities of the elderly. These cover such subjects as income, health services, housing, food and nutrition, transportation (access to health and medical care, church-cultural-recreation-social contacts), spiritual satisfaction, and life-long learning.

Another way to become attuned to the needs of our aging population is to ponder the "Declaration of Aging Rights" which arose from the 1971 White House Conference on Aging. Among the conditions of justice due our older or retired citizens, the Conference declared to be:

> 1. The right to live with sufficient means for decency and self-respect.
> 2. The right to move about freely, reasonably and conveniently.
> 3. The right to pursue a career or interest without penalty founded on age.
> 4. The right to be heard on all matters of general public interest.
> 5. The right to maintain health and well-being through preventive care and education.
> 6. The right to receive assistance in times of illness or need or other emergency.
> 7. The right to peace and privacy as well as participation.
> 8. The right to protection and safety amid the hazards of daily life.
> 9. The right to act together to seek redress of their grievances.
> 10. The right to live life fully and with honor — not for their age, but for their humanity (Baumann, 1971).

It should be readily apparent that the process of aging must concern everyone. It concerns the population between eighteen and sixty-five years of age since they must support the dependent, whether old or young. It concerns those under eighteen years of age "because the needs of the elderly compete for funds with needs for education and other services to youth" (Baumann, 1971).

REFERENCES

Baumann, Ruth: *Public and Private Partnership for Older Americans.* Madison, Institute of Governmental Affairs, University of Wisconsin-Extension, 1971.

deBeauvoir, Simone: *The Coming of Age.* New York, Putnam, 1972.

Fowler, Roy S. Jr., and Fordyce, Wilbert: Adapting care for the brain-damaged patient. *Am J Nurs, 72(11)*:2056, 1972.

Pincus, Allen: New findings on learning in old age: Implications for occuaptional therapy. *Am J Occup Ther, 22(4)*:300, 1968.

U.S. Department of Health, Education, and Welfare: *Working With Older People — A Guide to Practice, Vol. I: The Practitioner and the Elderly.* Washington, Public Health Service, 1969.

U.S. Department of Health, Education, and Welfare: *Working With Older People — A Guide to Practice, Vol. II: Biological, Psychological and Sociological Aspects of Aging.* Washington, Public Health Service, 1970.

ADDITIONAL READING LIST

Birren, James E. (Ed.): *Handbook of Aging and the Individual.* Urbana, U of Ill Pr, 1959.

Geist, Harold: *The Psychological Aspects of the Aging Process With Sociological Implications.* St. Louis, Green, 1968.

Kastenbaum, Robert: *New Thoughts on Old Age.* New York, Springer Pub, 1964.

Panegis, Constantine: Lectures on chronic disease and disability. University of Wisconsin-Extension, Health Sciences Unit, Feb. 25 and March 4, 1970.

Rodstein, Manuel: The aging process and disease. *Nurse Outlook, 12(11)*:43, 1964.

Shock, Nathan Wetheril: *Aging — Some Social and Biological Aspects.* Washington, American Association for the Advancement of Science, 1960.

U.S. Department of Health, Education, and Welfare: *Working With Older People — A Guide to Practice, Vol. III: The Aging Person: Needs and Services.* Washington, Public Health Service, 1970.

Zinberg, Norman E., and Kaufman, Irving: *Normal Psychology of the Aging Process.* New York, Intl Univs Pr, 1963.

Chapter 2

NURSING HOMES: ALTERNATIVES TO HOME AND HOSPITAL

A REVIEW of the literature on nursing homes introduces one to a full gamut of claims, hopes, petitions, achievements, and criticism. On the one hand we are told that people are sent to nursing homes to die (partly because the government "treated nursing home care as a housing, not a health program" (Pryor, 1970). Toward the other end of the continuum we are told that nursing homes of the future must "operate as a nonsurgical chronic disease hospital with psychiatric orientation in order to provide the dynamic patient services required by the chronically disabled. . . in which the functions of the therapeutic community are implemented by the services of all related professional disciplines — medicine, psychiatry, nursing, psychology, social work, physical therapy, occupational therapy, recreational therapy, and religious services — if full potential of patient rehabilitation is to be realized" (Miller,1966). Strangely enough, this latter, more encouraging, source omits speech pathology and audiology in its reference to *all* related professional disciplines.

This chapter attempts to describe some of the changing conditions affecting the daily life of cases or patients serviced by the various rehabilitation professions. To simplify matters, this discussion will group all home substitute settings — other than hospitals (acute, rehabilitation, psychiatric, and Veterans Administration) — under the generic term *nursing homes*. It seems futile to discuss in any great detail extended care facilities, intermediate care facilities, skilled nursing facilities, or any other type of home, the designations of which (as well as functions, population served, regulations, etc.) can prove to be quite transitory in response to national, regional, and local trends in health care. Many of the principles advanced in this book are of no less importance to present residential homes for the aged than they are to present *health halfway houses* — be they halfway from the hospital (for either acute of chronic disease) to the grave, or from the hospital back to the patient's own home.

A variety of factors have contributed to the proliferation of homes for the ill and aged. Not only is the average person's life span increasing, but concomitant changes in family living styles have made it impossible, or extremely difficult, for working wives to care for older relatives. Increasing hospital costs, and the concomitant (or resultant) development of nonhospital facilities, have created even greater demand for nursing homes. Not only is personal care required — i.e. room and board, plus help in walking and feeding — but skilled nursing and intensive care are also required.

In the midst of this demand, the various professions are still attempting to define operationally what is meant by *skilled nursing care*. Whatever it is, it is *not* mere custodial care (i.e. care designed to assist an individual to cope with his own activities of daily living). The Social Security Administration, as interpreted by the fiscal intermediary, cites three components of skilled nursing care. They are: (1) "professional observation and assessment of the total needs of the patient"; (2) "the act of planning, organization and management of a treatment plan involving multiple services where specialized health care knowledge must be applied"; and (3) "the rendering of direct services to a patient where the ability to provide the services requires specialized training" (Miller, 1970).

The pressures of the federal government to obtain better services for our chronically ill and aged have had repercussions that appear to include both good and bad aspects. A large number of private nursing homes came into existence because there was an excellent chance to *make a quick buck*. The government was more prompt in creating standards than it was in finding ways to enforce such standards. Enterprising businessmen saw opportunity in such a situation.

As highly verbal critics (including Ralph Nader) began to complain, the parties most concerned sought to regulate themselves and raise standards. A number of professional organizations came into being, such as The American Association of Homes for the Aging (for nonprofit institutions), The American Nursing Home Association (essentially for profit homes, but some nonprofits are included), and The American Hospital Association's section for long-term care institutions (under any sponsorship — nonprofit, proprietary, or governmental). In addition, The American Medical Association and The National Council for the Accreditation of Nursing Homes began to work toward setting national standards, to establish licensure procedures.

Also, in the effort to upgrade the quality of nursing home administration, the American College of Nursing Home Administrators was established in 1963. Regular membership requires completion of at least two years of training beyond high school plus successful completion of an oral or written examination prescribed by the board of governors. Associate membership requires at least three years' experience in long-term care, intention to continue in a career with long-term care institutions, and meeting requirements prescribed by the board of governors. An advanced type of membership is that of *Fellow*. This is open only to individuals with at least four years of acceptable training beyond high school, the publication of four articles on nursing homes (or completion of a fellowship project), and evidence of service beyond ordinary demands of his position. A list of fourteen objectives of the organization are presented in the November, 1967, article in *Professional Nursing Home* (pages 16 through 17) entitled "The Call to Professionalism in Administration."

The Social and Rehabilitation Services of the U.S. Dept. of Health, Education and Welfare created a set of "Recommended Rules and Regulations" (with guidelines) to guide State Licensing Boards of Nursing Home Administration. These regulations arose out of an extensive series of public hearings in major cities in 1968 and 1969. Along with the American Medical Association Council on Medical Service's "Report to the Secretary of HEW and the States," the guidelines form a foundation for levels of knowledge and experience desired for nursing home administrators to insure progressively higher quality nursing home patient care and education.

These various attempts to upgrade the quality of services undoubtedly will remain in a state of flux for some time, as will the overall subject of appropriate health care for the chronically ill and aged. During this period of upheaval and change, extreme variations from home to home, and from state to state, can be expected. The so-called retirement or rest homes, set up to provide custodial services incidental to aging, are attempting to accommodate the elderly with far more specialized needs. Some nursing homes are becoming nondistinguishable from subacute or chronic hospitals. Many states are discharging psychiatric patients to nonhospital settings such as nursing homes when no continued benefits are contemplated from continued service in mental hospitals.

The recognition of the need for rehabilitative efforts in nursing homes now widely permeates the pertinent literature. As early as 1967, Chafee designated staff education, patient motivation, and patient involvement in planning as the greatest needs in order to preserve patients' individuality and dignity. In a study of 223 patients in twenty-six licensed nursing homes in Massachusetts, Chafee found that more than 90 percent of the subjects were sixty-five years of age or older. The median age was eighty. He found that nearly 90 percent of the patients showed a significant hearing loss, that 19 percent needed further medical attention, that 12 percent needed regular physical therapy, that 4 percent needed occupational therapy, and that 92.5 percent needed special staff consideration with regard to speech and hearing. He further found 65 percent to have significant loss in motor tone and power, or in coordination. Visual deficits were judged *significant,* and well over one-third had a significant loss in dental function.

Many of the homes studied by Chafee did not know the history of the patients. With respect to physical therapy services, only six of the twenty-six homes had a physical therapy staff; nine drew upon the services of the Visiting Nurse Association, while the remaining had no physical therapy service. Registered occupational therapists were on the staff of only two homes, while unregistered *therapists* served at another two homes.

Out of this fact-finding experience, Chafee developed a series of recommendations based on a philosophy of rehabilitation. To implement such a philosophy would require staff education (professional and nonprofessional) in geriatric problems and in rehabilitation nursing care techniques, greater attention to the social and psychological needs of each patient, and *"continuous re-evaluation of the status and requirements of patients. . . . rather than indefinite continuation of initial services"* (Chafee, 1967). (Italics added by the author of this text, not that of the original author.)

The overall goal of *extended care,* as cited by Michael Miller (1970), is "to provide an alternative to hospital care for patients who still require general medical management and skilled nursing care on a continuing basis, but do not require the constant availability of physician services ordinarily found in a hospital setting." Mr. Miller also notes that "approval of an extended care facility as a Medicare provider of services requires a multidisciplinary rehabilitation team, including physicians, nurses, physical therapist, occupational therapy, speech therapist, recreation therapist, and social workers (Miller 1970).

It is apparent that those who care for the elderly must know more about personal adjustment and how to facilitate the resident's adjustment to his new home. This is a big order for most staffs whose training has been of a *traditional* type. For example, while physicians are presumed to be well-trained in diagnosis and pharmacological management, few of them are likely to have had much experience in the care of the ill aged.

Dr. Charles Kramer, psychiatric consultant to *Professional Nursing Home,* notes that "we have found it necessary to delve into many areas which we previously had thought were only tangential: the evolution of a therapeutic community, the understanding of communication processes, the significant emotional ties between psychologically related groups, the impact of interpersonal encounters, the significance of forces operating outside ordinary awareness, the crucial dependence upon an administrative matrix which intertwines intuition and knowledge in a highly sophisticated and sensitive way" (Kramer, 1968). Such a statement is far removed from any philosophy of nursing home management which remains solely disease-oriented.

Each successive year brings about an increase in the percentage of residents in each home who have histories of psychiatric illness. The net result is that the supervising nurse, who must coordinate all of the services, is now involved in psychosocial nursing. As is any charge nurse in a hospital, the supervising nurse in a nursing home must be aware of drugs prescribed and must be alert to the side effects of each resident's medication. Additionally, she participates in ongoing clinical diagnosis by alerting the physician to the possibility of undiagnosed diabetes, to bowel obstructions, congestive heart failure, fractures, etc. Her rehabilitation role keeps her involved in activities of daily living, bowel or bladder training, etc. She is involved in in-service training of the institution's staff. She may also be involved in facilitating training and research opportunities for outside training programs, such as for nursing, occupational therapy, speech pathology, and physical therapy. But above and beyond all these involvements, she is the one professional expected to facilitate the interpersonal relationships of each resident with his family, with other professionals, and with institutional personnel. To some nurses and to some institutions this last role is a relatively new one — the need to so interrelate with her residents or patients that their psychological, as well as physical, needs are served. She needs to detect significant behavioral change since often the patient cannot verbalize their problems because of "memory deficits, panic, agitation, confusion, disorientation as to time and place, and altered pain perception" (Miller, *et al.*, 1966).

How is this level of service to be accomplished — if at all? Obviously, the various educational institutions preparing professionals must overhaul their curricula. For present professionals, perhaps the best answer is in-service education similar to that in Illinois, reported by Nordstrom, and that in Wisconsin, reported by Jennerjohn.

Nordstrom describes a team which goes into selected licensed nursing homes throughout the state and works with and teaches personnel the philosophy and techniques of rehabilitation. The project, cited as "the first of its kind to be initiated in the U.S." (Nordstrom, 1963), has a physiatrist as its medical advisor, and utilizes teams composed of rehabilitation registered nurses and occupational therapists. Subjects included in their teaching, which continues for "as long as necessary' — i.e. from four to eight weeks — are the purpose of rehabilitation, the need for motivation, bowel and bladder training, principles of speech and hearing including problems of the aphasic patient, and demonstrations of passive and active range-of-motion exercises, pulley exercises, parallel bar exercises, body alignment and bed positioning, and transfer activities such as bed to chair.

Jennerjohn (1968) reported on in-service education institutes carried on by the state of Wisconsin's Section of Chronic Disease, and other sections of the division of health. He related that these institutes are intended to assist nursing homes in the area of rehabilitative nursing, recreational therapy, speech and hearing therapy, and nutrition and food services.

Nursing home programs benefitting from such activities are a far cry from disease-oriented care primarily interested in symptomatic relief.

One of the main problems experienced in achieving a rehabilitation environment in nursing homes is the matter of interest on the part of professionals — particularly the physician. Many doctors are easily discouraged when faced with clinical problems they cannot cure. Many are depressed by nursing home patients.

Need one have any doubts of the concern of the physician who encounters the following recommendation? "The physician should prepare the disabled worker psychologically and emotionally to accept compulsory retirement and adjustment if it is medically indicated... utilizing the... rehabilitation team ... to continue maintenance therapy... to achieve a gradual social and avocational adjustment to their new interpersonal relationships and new environmental circumstances,... (and) increase the independence, dignity, and self-respect of the individual" (Bova, 1967).

In the light of the reviving concept of family practice, future outlook on the function of physicians is most optimistic. It is hoped that a similarly optomistic spirit will infuse the ranks of the other professions whose services are so desparately needed in nursing homes and related institutions.

The burden placed upon personnel who seek to offer appropriate in-service training is enormous. It is readily apparent that the mere establishment of educational programs for nursing homes staffs does not equate to creating a therapeutic community. The mobility of personnel, even within the best-run institutions offering the best in-service programs, presents a constant challenge to the success of true team efforts. Work schedules involving each of the day's twenty-four hours present another major difficulty. Yet, if a true therapeutic community is to be achieved, it requires ongoing in-service training of *all* staff members — professional, lay people, volunteers.

Another potential detriment to success lies in exceeding the scope of authority of the in-service educators. Whether they be occupational therapists, physical therapists, speech pathologists, etc., these educators must accomplish their goals by giving instruction — not orders — to the staff.

In a true multidisciplinary approach, therapeutic goals and basic regimens of each specialist must be understood by all the other specialists. It is also possible for each professional to utilize various techniques of the other professions without violation of professional ethics. A speech pathology consultant, secure in his own professional knowledge, can help in achieving a community in which all disciplines participate in various ways and differing degrees in the language stimulation of poststroke patients. Staff guidance appears in varying degrees of specificity in this book, and in journal articles such as Jones and Kramer's 1967 article "Creating a Therapeutic Language Atmosphere." In using these (and other) sources, the avoidance of unethical staff activities and the improvement of patients are best assured by person-to-person discussions with speech pathologists, resident or consulting, on facilitating techniques and on contraindications of pursuing such techniques.

Numerous publications have cited patients' or residents' *needs*. We read that "food, clothing, shelter and medical services are not enough. The overall continued well-being of the patient necessarily is connected intimately with his feelings, attitudes, emotions, drives, and motivations.... the patient has a series of continuing needs. He has a need to feel and be clean, be listened to, be useful and needed. He has an ongoing need to give and to receive. He has a need to communicate with others and tell of his wants. He has to satisfy these needs and, hopefully, achieve satisfying new experiences. In short, many patients need emotional prophylaxis...He has a need for self-expression, a need to have something to do, a need to have companionship in the doing" (Routh, 1967).

Attempts to contend with these needs have led to a variety of techniques of approaches such as *activity therapy* and *milieu* (environment) *therapy*. In such contexts, a physically healthy but inactive person is just as nonfunctional and *sick* as a person invalided by disease. Activity therapy, accordingly, embraces various techniques of work, recreation, education, and physical treatment. Such therapy demands a realistic encounter with one's surroundings. Meaningful exchange must be maintained with others and with the environment.

In contrast to the ideation involved in the *disengagement theory,* social contacts, productive work, and education characterize normal and successful aging. Good adjustment and mental health are associated with continued activity, interest, and contact with other people. Increased socialization is achieved through verbal interaction. *Activity therapy* postulates that vivid stimulation, continued challenge, productivity, and, in particular, group interaction, contributes in special ways to the health of older persons. On the other hand, contributors to chronic depression include restraint of convalescent confinement, lack of mobility, and *protective custody* of a sheltering institution (Davis, 1967).

A related technique, or approach, is that of *milieu therapy*. The person's total social milieu is utilized as an instrument of treatment. Paramount is all of the patient's activities, and all of his interactions with the staff and with other patients. Interactions are observed, analyzed, and discussed until understood. Such an approach forces patients and staff to work together and requires a constant focus on communication.

Awareness of roles, responsibilities, and relationships creates a team attitude. The openness introduced between all parties minimizes misunderstanding and conflict among staff and patients. Greater mutual understanding comes about. *Feeling tone* of a floor of patients becomes sensed by the staff. The *difficult* resident gets better handling. While such positive gains are claimed for the practice of milieu therapy in nursing homes by a psychiatrist (see Grauer, 1971), the present author notes the emphasis on communication — listening and speaking — on all levels, as a key to therapy. Dr. Grauer's article cites the need for respect and realistic goals in caring for and living with aged residents. As such, it is an account of value to anyone serving nursing homes as staff members or as volunteers.

Dr. Grauer's article might be profitably studied, particularly in view of the apparently nationwide exodus of less acutely ill psychiatric patients from mental hospitals to nursing homes. One of the results of this trend, according to Collins, Stotsky, and Dominick is that the nursing home is becoming "like the back ward of the custodial mental hospitals of the past." With routinization conformity and lack of contact with professionals, patients tend to become stereotyped, their individual identity gets submerged, they are cared for by an untrained (in psychiatric techniques) staff, and their dignity and self-worth are destroyed. Collins, Stotsky, and Dominick note that "although the majority of patients in nursing homes, regardless of their prior medical history, show significant psychiatric pathology, psychiatric resources are not readily available to most nursing homes" (Collins, *et al.*, 1967). The same statement might just as correctly be made concerning speech pathology and communication problems. Despite discrepancies between the ideal and the actual, nursing homes must continue to satisfy the customer, relatives, hospital personnel, welfare caseworkers, and the public health inspector.

REFERENCES

Bova, Alexander W.: The physician's responsibility in using a rehabilitation concept in his treatment of the aging: In nursing homes and extended care facilities. In Margolin, Reuben J., and Goldin, George (Eds.): *Dynamic Programming in the Rehabilitation of the Aging*. Boston, Dept. of Rehabilitation and Special Education, Northeastern University; Washington, D.C., U.S. Dept. of Health, Education and Welfare, 1967.

Chafee, Charles E.: Rehabilitation needs of nursing home patients — a report of a survey. *Rehabil Lit, 28(12)*:377, 1967.

Collins, Jerome A., Stotsky, Bernard A., and Dominick, Joan R.: Is the nursing home the mental hospital's back ward in the community? *J Am Geriatr Soc., 15(1)*:75, 1967.

Davis, Robert William: Activity therapy in a geriatric setting. *J Am Geriatr Soc, 15(12)*:1144, 1967.

Grauer, H.: Institutions for the aged — therapeutic communities? *J Am Geriatr Soc, 19(8)*:687, 1971.

Jennerjohn, Dale: Impact of Medicare and Medicaid on nursing home development. *Health, 18(5)*:21, 1968.

Jones, Wendell E., and Kramer, Charles H.: Creating a therapeutic language atmosphere. *Professional Nurs Home, 9(9)*:46, 1967.

Kramer, Charles H.: Twenty years of nursing home changes. *Professional Nurs Home, 10(3)*: 24, 1968.

Miller, Michael B.: The nursing home, society, and the law. *Geriatrics, 21(3)*:193, 1966.

Miller, Michael B.: Phasing out Medicare: Changing definitions of skilled nursing care and custodial care. *J Am Geriatr Soc, 18(12)*:937, 1970.

Miller, Michael B., Keller, Dorothy, Liebel, Eduard, and Meirowitz, Irene: Nursing in a skilled nursing home. *Am J Nurs, 66(2)*:321, 1966.

Nordstrom, Margene J.: Rehabilitating the care in nursing homes. *Am J Nurs, 63(2)*:101, 1963.

Pryor, David H.: Somewhere between society and the cemetery: where we put the aged. *The New Republic, 162*:15, April 25, 1970.

Routh, Thomas A.: What's your philosophy? *Professional Nurs Home, 9(11)*:36, 1967.

ADDITIONAL READING LIST

Allen, Rex Whitaker: Nursing homes. *Architectural Record, 142(10)*:¹£&[¹&¢%]

Anderson, Helen: Rehabilitation — a new emphasis in nursing home care. *Rehabil Rec, 4(4)*:30, 1963.

Anonymous: Austin volunteers provide services for nursing home patients. *Aging, 168*:8, Oct-Nov, 1968.

Anonymous: The call to professionalism in administration. *Professional Nurs Home, 9(11)*:16, 1967.

Anonymous: Nader v. Nursing Homes. *Time, 96(4)*:48, 1970.

Anonymous: What to look for in a nursing home. *Today's Health, 45(9)*:84, 1967.

Bloomer, H. Harlan: Communication problems among aged county hospital patients. *Geriatrics, 15(4)*:291, 1960.

Derman, Sheila, and Manaster, Albert: Family counseling with relatives of aphasic patients at Schwab Rehabilitation Hospital. *ASHA, 9(5)*:175, 1967.

Foxhall, William B.: New legislation puts fresh impetus behind nursing homes and housing for the elderly. *Achitectural Record, 139(6)*:151, 1966.

Gordon, Helen G., and McTavey, Harriet E.: Relationship between past and present activity of female residents in a geriatric home. *J Am Geriatr Soc, 17(5)*:493, 1969.

Greenwald, Shayna, and Linn, Margaret W.: What wives say about nursing homes. *J Am Geriatr Soc, 18(2)*:166, 1970.

Kelly, Trubie: Operational problems in the nursing home. *Hospital Management, 100(5)*:94, 1965.

Kramer, Charles H., and Kramer, Jeannette R.: The nursing home as a total therapeutic situation: Some basic assumptions. *J Geriatr Psychiatry, 1(2)*:179, 1968.

Kramer, Charles H., and Petersen, Lucille S.: A volunteer's discussion group. *Professional Nurs Home, 9(5)*42, 1967.

Linn, Margaret W.: A nursing home rating scale. *Geriatrics, 21(10)*:188, 1966.

Miller, Michael B.: Changing perspectives and cross-currents in nursing home care, 1968-1969. *J Am Geriatr Soc, 18(2)*: 176, 1970a.

Miller, Michael B.: Medical care in the extended care facility. *J Am Geriatr Soc, 19(2)*:102, 1971.

Miller, Michael B.: Physical, emotional and social rehabilitation in a nursing-home population. *J Am Geriatr Soc, 13(2)*:176, 1965.

Pastore, John O., Winston, Frederick B., Barrett, Harold S., and Foote, Franklin, M.: Characteristics of patients and medical care in New Haven area nursing homes. *N Engl J med, 279(3)*:130, 1968.

Pugnier, Vincent A., and Jordan, William A.: Gerodontal problems in Minnesota's chronic care facilities. *Northwest Dentistry, 50*:21, 1971.

Randall, Ollie A.: The situation with nursing homes. *Am J Nurs, 65(11)*:92, 1965.

Remily, Louis: Nursing home care under Medicare. *Health, 18(1)*:7, 1967.

Schober, William R.: A successful rehab program. *Professional Nurs Home, 10(1)*:19, 1968.

Swaim, William T., Jr.: The ideal administrator. *Professional Nurs Home, 10(10*:28, 1968.

Walle, Eugene L., and Newman, Parley W.: Rehabilitation services for speech, hearing, and language disorders in an extended care facility. *ASHA*, 9(6):216, 1967.

Weiss, Curtis E.: Communicative needs of the geriatric population. *J Am Geriatr Soc, 19(7)*:640, 1971.

Chapter 3

THE TEAMWORK TREND IN HEALTH CARE DELIVERY

INTERPROFESSIONAL *teamwork*... In the past few years this expression has been heard with ever-increasing frequency. Seldom, however, do the people who speak or write this expression indicate the referents or connotations intended. There seems to be a tacit assumption that this expression has similar meanings to all people. The author seriously questions such an assumption.

Within the profession of speech pathology and audiology the concept of interprofessional teamwork has been steadily advanced. Again, even within this circumscribed population, it is questionable to what extent two users of the expression would hold identical meanings therefore. For example, much is said about interprofessional teamwork occurring in medical settings. Presumably this concept is championed on the assumption that all members will work on an equal level, and group decisions with respect to cases will be made as a result of the democratic process.

Is the idea of *team* a particularly democratic concept? The 1966 unabridged edition of the *Random House Dictionary of the English Language* indicates that a team is "a number of persons associated in some joint action, especially one of the sides in a game or contest" (Stein, 1966). One of the definitions of *team* in *Webster's Third New International Dictionary* is "a number of persons associated together in work or activity as a group of specialists or scientists functioning as a collaborative unit." However, sports-conscious Americans are more apt to associate the word with a different Webster definition — i.e. "a number of persons selected to contend on one side in a match (as in cricket, football, rowing, or a debate") (Gove, 1971)

While these and other definitions from various dictionaries

suggest some type of cooperative effort, I would seriously question whether this is the intent of some of our colleagues in speech and hearing, as well as some of our colleagues of other health-related professions, when they talk about *teamwork.*

If teams are headed by captains, then we might briefly look at two definitions of "captain." The *Random House Dictionary* cites "a person who is at the head of or in authority over others" (Stein, 1966). The *Webster Third* lists "a person having authority over and responsibility for a group or unit," and "a leader of a side or team in a sports contest or similar activity" (Gove, 1971).

In the world of sports a team is captained by one individual whose relationship to the other team members is seldom that of equality. The captain directs, leads, and is responsible for team actions. The captain is at the head of, or in authority over, others. Such functions would seem to preclude the concept of equal participation. If use of the word *team* by members of professions allied to health embraces the concept of a captain, then I think we had better give just recognition to whom we are willing to have captain this team, and stop talking about teamwork as if it is all a matter of equality of all members of the team. If, on the other hand, we truthfully do not wish to have our teams captained, with the resultant jockeying for leadership position, perhaps we should cease using the word *team* and use instead the word *consortium* — i.e. "any association, partnership, or union" (Stein, 1966).

Possibly such distinctions are merely academic. Present-day tradition and practices recognize that the physician is legally responsible for the case's well-being. However, this legal responsibility should not be confused with the moral responsibility of the speech pathologist to determine *how* to treat communication problems.

Regardless of the amount of power structure of various teams, it is widely believed that we can all learn by participation in (so-called) team efforts. Presuming that the team is patient-focused, rather than discipline-centered, each person can make his unique contribution to the team itself, as well as to patient care. Each professional can become a collaborator, a consultant, a teacher.

A major challenge facing the health-related professions is to find new ways for adapting our categorical and specialist-centered resources to the needs of people through comprehensive, family-centered care. Ideally each team member must be knowledgeable in the broad aspects of the other professions involved. Such knowledge is acquired through resolving case-handling disagreements, while demonstrating respect for others' competence, as well as fallibility. As we move toward a mastery of overlapping bodies of knowledge directed toward total person adjustment, each specialist also moves toward a consultant function. Ideal teamwork requires a reciprocal give and take for the patient's good. Such interplay can only be based on a respect for the opinions of one's co-workers, plus recognition that no one discipline is more important than the other — no one "owns" the patient. Each person representing a given profession needs recognition, not awe.

Let us take a look at four major *teams* with which speech pathology has traditionally identified. (This discussion is best understood when one realizes that in America, speech pathology evolved through the profession of education, rather than through medicine).

Within the school system there is the congregation of specialists assembled in orthopedic schools, particularly for the purpose of meeting the needs of cerebral palsied children. There was seldom any question within this type of group effort as to whether or not a team leader or captain was desired. Certainly, if for no other reason, the team was relieved to have one of its members assume full legal responsibility for any adverse effects of any of the various treatments which might be administered to the child.*

Another team was that organized by speech clinicians around the so-called *secondary* stutterer.† The assistance of parents, grandparents, teacher, coach, clergyman, interested neighbors, etc., was solicited. By no stretch of the imagination was it ever

---

*An older but less formal public school *team* is the classic interrelationship of the speech clinician and the classroom teacher.

†Kenneth Scott Wood, in his glossary of terms used in speech pathology and audiology, defines secondary stuttering as "neuromuscular spasms of the speech mechanism accompanied by anxiety about nonfluency and accompanied by habitual irrelevant movements used as devices to break up or conceal speech blockages" (Kenneth Scott Wood, "Terminology and Nomenclature," in Travis, Lee Edward (ed.), *Handbook of Speech Pathology and Audiology*, New York, Appleton-Century-Crofts, 1971, p. 19).

considered for one moment that this group of individuals would proceed in any type of therapeutic assistance without guidance through counseling, if not outright direction, by the speech clinician captaining this team.

Another type of team has been that of the various experts who organized themselves in mutual concern for young aphasic adults. This type of team developed, primarily in Veterans Administration Hospitals, through approaches to the rehabilitation of young aphasic adults during and following World War II.

A fourth type of team has been that of the group of specialists who direct their attention to the study and treatment of individuals having a cleft lip, cleft palate, or other orofacial anomaly. Again, the *team* idea seems inevitably to foster a jockying for position of captaincy of that team.

As a preliminary to analyzing the teamwork concept's potential effectiveness, the author had the students in his graduate course, "The Speech Pathologist's Role with the Chronically Ill and Aged," evolve a list of professions represented on *teams* with which they were familiar. The composition of this class, in terms of where they received their previous education, frees the resultant list from the possible parochialism of a single community or state. Table I tabulates composite team memberships cited by the students, deleting identifying reference to any specific Milwaukee- or Wisconsin-based teams.

The author found this information as instructive for the personnel omitted as for those professions which were included. The clergy and family members (in this case, parents) were each represented on only one of these teams. The patient himself was missing from all of the teams. These omissions are singularly interesting and symptomatic of some of our problems.

Subsequent probing of these same students for lists of team membership deemed *typical* in homes for the aged revealed the following: director of the home, eye specialists (ophthalmologists and opticians), geriodontist, nutritionist, nurses, nurses' aides, occupational therapist, physical therapist, and physician (general practitioner), as well as podiatrist. Again, neither clergy, family, nor the patient himself were mentioned.

Table I

TEAMWORK

	Cleft Palate Team	*Acute Hospital Based Rehabilitation Team*	*V.A. Hospital Based Rehabilitation Team*	*Public School Diagnostic (Child Study) Center*
Audiologist	X	X	X	X
Clergyman		X		
Dentistry				
Pedodontist	X			
Orthodontist	X			
Prosthodontist	X			
Educational Therapist			X	
Family (parents, spouse)				X
Geneticist	X			
Nurse	X	X	X	X
Nutritionist	X	X		
Occupational Therapist		X	X	
Physical Therapist		X	X	
Physician				
Geneticist	X			
Laryngologist	X			
Neurologist			X	
Otologist	X			
Pediatrician	X			X
Physiatrist		X		
Plastic Surgeon	X			
Psychiatrist			X	
Radiologist	X			
Psychologist	X		X	X
Social Worker	X	X	X	X
Speech Pathologist	X	X	X	X
School Personnel				
Principal				X
Classroom Teacher				X
Guidance Specialist				X
Reading Specialist				X
Social Worker				X
Special Education Teacher				X
Speech Pathologist				X
Vocational Rehabilitation Specialist			X	

The author interprets the absence of the patient from these lists as indicative of *depersonalization of the patient.* In many, if not most, instances, should not the adult patient be a member of the team? Should he not help set his own goals since he is partly responsible for his own recovery?

Far too frequently, the members of a team see and report upon the patient's problems serially. They make suggestions or recommendations to other professionals. The medical social worker sums up. Then the physician decides — with or without the pooled information available — and determines priorities. Such procedures can give rise to interdepartmental and interprofessional conflict with each professional acting completely on his own. Unnecessary duplication occurs due to overlap; appropriate conclusions are not arrived at; follow-up recommendations are absent or ambiguous; the family does not understand; original diagnostic *labeling* may be clung to without modification despite contesting or conflicting evidence; etc.

Frequently the matter of professional overlap gives rise to fears, resentments, and defensiveness about *our territory.* On the other hand, it is in precisely these areas of overlap where professional insight and learning is most apt to occur — when professionals determine common and realistic goals utilizing shared information.

Within the past decade there has been an increasing concern for the older adult. This concern is fostering still more references to team efforts, particularly in rehabilitation departments or centers attempting to rehabilitate adults with impaired communication abilities — be they in their middle years or be they members of the so-called geriatric, or over sixty-five, group.

How can health-related professionals effectively work together in achieving better adjustment of their middle-aged and aging clients who have experienced communication breakdowns? Let us examine the possible role of the speech and hearing clinician in the total rehabilitation effort involved in dealing with our communication-impaired aging and aged populations. To deal effectively with communication disorders, speech and hearing personnel are necessarily thrown into close work with members of the professions sometimes referred to as paramedical professions, in addition to the professions of medicine, dentistry, and the law. Any effective input to group effort can only be achieved if the professional relates effectively within the total rehabilitation plan, if he understands his co-workers who are involved and interrelating with the case.

As the profession of speech pathology and audiology developed in the United States, the phrase *the whole child* became a crusading by-line. University and college programs training speech and hearing clinicians to work with children made extensive efforts to school the would-be clinician in various aspects of understanding the child within his environment. Not only did this require that the speech pathologist be familiar with the normal development of speech, hearing, and language, and abberations thereof, but that he also be familiar with philosophies of education, the history of education in this country, and with awarenesses of the child in relationship to his school and his society. Training programs began to require more and more courses which enabled the would-be clinician to understand the ways in which his professional efforts would be aided, or could be aided and abetted, as he dealt with his client in the broader contexts of his home, his school, his neighborhood, his state, and his nation. These general ideas have acquired such credence and acceptance that it would probably be impossible to locate training programs which operate oblivious to the larger ramifications of communication breakdowns within society.

However, it would appear that not all speech and hearing training programs have exerted the same care in studying cases in relationship to their total environment when dealing with mature adults as they have when dealing with the growing child. Is it at all possible for speech and hearing clinicians to work effectively with older adult populations without having a good solid understanding of the aging individual, his physical and physiological changes, his emotional changes, the reactions to a changing society, and his changing roles within that changing society? Should not the profession of speech pathology and audiology be as equally careful in training clinicians to work with the older adult as it has been in training clinicians to work with the young child?

This is not advanced as a purely rhetorical question. The substance of this entire book is a partial answer to this question. It is a plea that those who profess to be capable of working with the communication problems of the aging and the aged acquire the information and competencies necessary to do this job. Such an approach requires a broad knowledge of the training and competencies of all those individuals involved in seeking to provide the best possible patient care.

The speech and hearing clinician must understand the complexities of the role expectations of nurses, for example. He must be aware of the competencies and ethical limitations of the various professions such as occupational therapy, physical therapy, dentistry, physiatry, psychiatry, psychology, social work, rehabilitation counseling. The list is long. The effectiveness of his interrelationship with individuals from all of these professions will strongly affect the extent and type of professional expectations that can be made of them.

By the same token, his efficiency will be helped or hindered by the extent to which members of those professions understand his competencies and limitations. An examination of professional training and treatment roles appears in a later chapter of this book.

REFERENCES

Gove, Philip Babcock (Ed.): *Webster's Third New International Dictionary of the English Language*. Springfield, Merriam, 1971.

Stein, Jess (Ed.): *The Random House Dictionary of the English Language*. New York, Random, 1966.

Chapter 4

HEARING

ACOUSTIC PROPERTIES OF SOUND

IN order to comprehend some of the problems experienced in understanding the spoken word, particularly as this understanding is interfered with by aging and various disease processes, it is necessary to have at least an elementary knowledge of the acoustical properties of speech sounds. The next few paragraphs attempt to simplify this information as much as possible. They try to make meaningful what must otherwise remain perplexing mysteries to the person encountering unusual responses of the hard-or-hearing to the spoken word.

The acoustic element easiest to understand is that of *loudness*. Most people react to a person's having difficulty in understanding by talking louder. For some individuals, this is sufficient. The listener's sound acuity (the keenness or sharpness of his hearing) achieves adequacy with an increase in the loudness of the speech signal. While this might suffice for some individuals, increased loudness is frequently insufficient for improving speech reception of other hard-of-hearing people.

Another generally understood concept is that of *pitch* — the highness or lowness of a sound on the musical scale. We react to the ups and downs of the melodic patterns of spoken speech. Extreme deviations from the normal rise and fall of the speaking voice can result in adverse listener reaction. For example, a person whose voice seldom changes in pitch level is said to speak in a *monotone*. The average listener, even though he may not identify the difference as a monotone, is apt to perceive the monotonous speaker as a dull, uninteresting person. Similarly, many people tend to have relatively stereotyped reactions to the woman who consistently speaks at too low a pitch level, or the man who consistently speaks at too high a pitch level.

An awareness solely of these differences in pitch and loudness is insufficient knowledge for the professional worker dealing with the chronically ill and aged. Let us analyze these factors, along with other acoustic phenomena, in somewhat greater depth.

The concept of sound is integrally associated with the concept of vibration. Dependent upon one's frame of reference, one might say that sound *is* vibration; or one might say that sound *results from* vibration (i.e. sound is vibration which is perceived by the listener). In either case, we need to know more about the properties of sound. Increased understanding is normally centered around the four concepts of pitch, loudness, quality, and duration.

Pitch

Most of us who are not tone deaf have at least a vague sort of idea of the pitch of sounds. When we sing or play a musical instrument, we talk about producing middle C, or D, or E flat, etc. We know that if we focus our voice at a given point on the musical scale, we can check our pitch by hitting the keys on the piano until we find the note that we are most closely approximating. When we sing a melody, we say that we are producing a standardized sequence of notes — each of which has a definite pitch.

The matter of highness or lowness on the musical scale is chiefly related to (or is the direct outcome of) the frequency at which the sound source is vibrating. Other things being equal, the faster the vibration, the higher the frequency, or perceived pitch. The slower the vibration, the lower the pitch. When the vibrating agent oscillates at a regular rate, the resultant sound is *periodic*. This property enables the hearer to assign a pitch level to the sound. Sounds which do not have this periodicity or repetition of vibrational pattern are called *aperiodic* sounds or *noise*. The piercing sound occasionally created in scratching a piece of chalk over a chalkboard is an example of what most of us call noise. The hissing of steam is another. In speech, we make a good number of these aperiodic sounds, but instead of calling them noise, we call them *voiceless* sounds — i.e. speech sounds made without the periodic vibration of the vocal folds.

Generally speaking, we talk of two main classes of voiceless sounds. One type results from a tiny explosion (or rapid release) of momentarily-damned up air. The *stop* sounds normally associated with the letters "p," "t," and "k" are examples. The other main class of voiceless sounds is that resulting from the turbulence of air being forced through narrowly-constricted passageways momentarily formed by our oral mechanism. These sounds (s, f, sh, etc.) are called *fricatives.*

We also use speech sounds which incorporate both periodic vibration *and* aperiodic turbulence. Examples would be sounds associated with the spelling "z," "v," etc. (See Appendix A for a chart of the sounds used in American English, listed in symbols of the International Phonetic Alphabet.)

Although the human ear cannot assign a pitch level to the voiceless sounds, laboratory equipment is capable of recording and measuring the pitch ranges at which vibration occurs during such sounds. A review of the sound measurement literature quickly reveals that much of the power of these voiceless sounds is concentrated in frequency ranges far higher than the characteristic levels at which the voiced (vocal fold vibration) sounds are made. The perception of such sounds demands hearing mechanisms capable of reacting to pitch levels far higher than those usually associated with vowel sounds and voiced consonants. Indeed, we realize that the flow of speech includes rapidly changing peaks and valleys of pitch, requiring hearing sensitivity over a considerable frequency range.

One of the characteristics of the aging person's hearing is that acuity for the higher pitches becomes less and less effective, ultimately narrowing the frequency range to which one is capable of responding. The *normal adult ear* can respond to a wide range of frequencies — frequently cited as ranging from sixteen or twenty cycles per second to 16,000 to 20,000 cycles per second. The term *cycles per second,* recently supplanted by the term *Hertz,* refers to the number of complete vibrations occurring during each second. Thus the middle C on the piano results from a vibration of approximately 256 Hertz (previously 256 cycles per second, or 256~).

As the aging ear becomes incapable of reacting to the higher frequencies, there is a continuing change in the perceived *quality* of sound, as well as an eventual inability to hear the high frequency speech sounds such as the voiceless "th" (as in "thumb"), the "s," and the "f." Normally, an increase in loudness will not enable the listener with such high frequency loss to hear the missing sounds. Hearing aids are of limited help in compensating for this type of loss. Such high frequency loss is characteristic of *presbycusis* — "the diminution of hearing acuity associated with old age" (Travis, 1971).

With the progressive inability to hear various speech sounds, the total flow of speech begins to lose its intelligibility for us. If medical and surgical treatment, along with hearing aid fitting, proves useless, we need other means to bolster our diminishing abilities for communication — such as speechreading (formerly known as lipreading). This avenue of supplementation may also become unavailable or useless as our sense of vision becomes increasingly more impaired.

Loudness

The element of *loudness* is most closely associated with the acoustic property of *intensity*. Sounds with a great deal of intensity are perceived as loud; sounds with little intensity are perceived as soft or weak. Our individual speech sounds have characteristically different intensity levels. The rapidly fluctuating loudness levels of individual speech sounds, in addition to a person's characteristic overall loudness level, play a significant role in the hearing of speech. Intensity is measured in units called *decibels* (dB). The decibel scale is a ratio scale, rather than one of *equal-intervals* such as the ruler incorporates. The human ear accommodates a range of approximately 120 decibels, from the just barely audible sound to sounds that cause pain to the ear.

When an individual suffers a hearing loss that affects all frequencies relatively equally, the loss is most frequently identified as a *conductive loss*. A conductive loss suggests that the causal factor will be something that is impeding the progress of the sound to the inner ear and brain. Such impedance might be due to impacted wax on the eardrum, minimizing the effectiveness of sound transmission into the middle ear. It might be due to impaired functioning of the three tiny bones in the middle ear — bones which convey the mechanical movements of the eardrum to the inner ear.

Once the cause of hearing loss is attributable to pathology in the inner ear and/or the nerve of hearing (eighth cranial nerve), one can no longer speak of a conductive loss, but of a *sensorineural loss.*

Conductive losses are more apt to be reversible than sensorineural losses. They can yield most successfully to the medical services or the operative techniques of an ear specialist. Individuals with sensorineural losses may or may not be assisted by amplification.

Quality

The element of sound known as *quality* is somewhat more difficult to explain and to understand. In speaking of a person's tone quality, we refer to the pleasantness or unpleasantness of the sounds uttered. Various qualities are referred to as *breathy, nasal, hoarse,* etc. The judgment implied in such labeling — strongly culturally influenced — is based on the components that make up the sound. To grasp this concept it is necessary to realize that the human larynx is incapable of producing a so-called *pure tone,* i.e. one comprised of vibration at a single frequency. Instead, the complexity of vocal fold vibration gives rise to many frequencies occurring simultaneously. In as simple a task as sustaining a vowel sound, the total amount of acoustic power is divided throughout a fairly wide range of the frequency spectrum. Various *bands* of frequency are produced at the same time, each with a different amount of sound power.

The lowest frequency at which a concentration of sound power is present is called the *fundamental frequency*. It is this frequency level which helps us to identify the pitch of a given sound. When we identify a given note or level on the musical scale, we are reacting primarily to the fundamental frequency.

However, the ear does not *zero in* on this frequency level at the expense of all the other frequencies present. It does not *turn off* the other (higher) frequencies. Instead, these additional sounding frequencies (overtones) are perceived as a part of the whole tone. They comprise the wave composition of the sound, which we react to when we talk about the quality of the tone, i.e. the pleasantness or unpleasantness of the sound. The closer these simultaneously-sounding frequency bands are to arithmetic multiples of the fundamental frequency, the better the tone quality — the more *pleasing* the sound. The further these higher frequencies are from multiples of the fundamental, the more likely we are to refer to the resultant sound as noise, i.e. frequencies sounding indiscriminately over the frequency range, with no apparent pattern of multiples.

The overall quality of a voice results from a composite of the complexity of vocal fold vibration, coupled with the interaction of the various cavities through which the vibrated airstream must pass — the throat, mouth, and/or nose. In the process of *resonance,* the changing size and shapes of the cavities, along with the size and shapes of the orifices (i.e. back of mouth, front of mouth, and nostril openings) modify the wave composition by amplifying some overtones at the expense of others which are *dampened,* or diminished, in power. Hence, the quality of speech depends upon the integrity and health of the total speech pathway from the larynx on out.

Another vital factor is that of respiration, which makes possible the speech sounds in the first place. Any physical or physiological deviations of the respiratory-oral tract — be they insufficiency of tissue, paralysis, paresis, etc. — can have an effect upon the distribution of sound power in the acoustic spectrum. Consequent redistribution of sound power will affect the quality of sound produced.

Similarly, from the standpoint of reception, deficiencies of the hearing mechanism will affect the signal received. The example of high fidelity record players illustrates this matter. Records from the early days of 78 rpm (revolutions per minute) recordings sound strange (*tinny, thin, poor* in quality) even when played upon the best reproducing equipment. This is primarily due to the restricted frequency ranges of the equipment used in producing the records. Inability to hear the higher overtones created by the musicians in the recording studio affects our reaction to the sounds' quality. A contemporary hi-fi record capable of producing undistorted overtones up to 20,000 Hz sounds natural — without distortion — if our hearing is relatively normal. As we lose more and more higher frequencies in the aging process, the best hi-fi recordings ultimately begin to sound similar to those early 78's.

Because of the overtone range of the instruments concerned, one would expect to hear the greatest distortion of the violins, cymbals, oboes, and clarinets — all of which produce overtones above 10,000 Hz. In terms of the fundamental pitches themselves, a person with presbycusis would expect to completely lose first the piccolo and then the upper ranges of the violins and flutes, as his hearing of the higher frequencies deteriorates.

One might question the recording deficiencies. In the case of the earliest recordings it was a matter of acquiring electronic know-how. In the case of later equipment it became a matter of cost. The greater the undistorted frequency response of any piece of reproducing equipment, the greater the cost.

We can adjust to the slow incipient changes in our perception of music. Most of us *cannot* adjust graciously as individual speech sounds begin to fade and disappear because of the consequent loss in intelligibility.

Duration

A fourth element of sound is that of duration. This word is used in its general sense. When we think of abnormally long durations, such as are encountered at times in the sound prolongations of stutterers, and when we also think of the related concept of *rhythm,* we can begin to perceive that time aspects of speech (duration of pauses as well as of vocalization) can become problems, particularly in persons suffering neurological disorders.

In summary, the properties of frequency (pitch), intensity (loudness), wave composition (quality), and duration play a vital role in speech. Disruptions of any of these factors can result in problems for the person so affected and for his listeners. All such problems can be augmented and aggravated by various psychosocial states and degenerations.

AUDITION AND AUDIOLOGICAL TESTING

Of the traditional five senses, those of hearing and vision are the most directly involved in communication. Vision is a major avenue of communication input. Most of us are reasonably familiar with, and can readily understand, the communication deficits due to farsightedness, nearsightedness, astigmatism, glaucoma, the development of cataracts, etc. Probably far less understood, and certainly far less apparent to the average person, are the poststroke problems arising from visual field cuts. These are dealt with in greater detail in the chapter on stroke. In the case of the blind, the sense of touch can be of vital importance in receiving messages, particularly by the braille technique of reading. As they age, the blind need procedures designed to preserve their skills of touch. Physical therapists and occupational therapists can reasonably be expected to play a role in such maintenance therapy.

However, it is the sense of hearing, more than any of the other senses, which is most closely related to the average person's lifelong skills of communication. The least sophisticated observer is acutely aware of the heroic efforts required of the person born deaf to learn to speak. Yet many of us are unaware of behavioral clues which suggest the possibility of less severe hearing deficiencies. The following list of patient behaviors is based on information obtained primarily from nurses who have indicated that this kind of information, which they feel is mandatory for nurses, was not part of their own training programs. Observable patient behaviors which suggest possible hearing problems include the following.

1. Frequent responses of *a-hum*
2. Apparent confusion
3. Responds better in quiet than in noise
4. Unable to satisfactorily converse on the telephone

5. Consistently speaks too loud
6. Speaks consistently at too soft a loudness level
7. Has vertigo problems (dizziness)
8. Has pain in his ear(s)
9. Has discharge from his ear(s)
10. Uses speech which is not readily intelligible
11. Appears withdrawn, detached from the environment
12. Appears to rely on facial expression for understanding the spoken word

The doctor and/or the patient's family should be contacted with reference to suspected hearing loss. The family will appreciate being acquainted with the pertinent community resources (frequently listed in community resource directories). Services invariably are available to anyone who cáres enough to find out where they are. Otologists and certified audiologists are the professionals best prepared to help regain or retain the best hearing possible. These specialists devote their careers to measuring and coping with alterations in hearing abilities.

This book does not purport to deal with all the intricate problems faced by these two professional groups in their daily professional activities. Instead, it selectively draws upon the vast corpus of information available in the hope of assisting health-related professionals to better cope with patient problems which arise from hearing handicaps.

Berger and Millin (1971) stress the need to understand the sometimes overlapping roles of the otologist, the audiologist, and the hearing aid dealer. They state:

> The roles of the otologist, audiologist, and hearing aid dealer should be clear, although these roles sometimes overlap. The otologist is responsible for diagnosing the hearing impairment and the medical or surgical treatment of the ear. The audiologist makes available to the physician audiologic diagnostic test results for the overall medical diagnosis. The audiologist also evaluates the patient's need for amplification and, if indicated, determines the approximate instrument requirements for the individual. He also has the responsibility of directing the overall aural rehabilitation of the patient. The hearing aid dealer is responsible for the precise fitting of the aid and its earmold, selling it, servicing it, and for helping the

individual to adjust to amplification when no great problems are encountered" (Berger and Millin, 1971).

The clinical audiologist, working closely with the otologist, helps to determine the best course of action. Frequently speechreading (lipreading) is the best solution. However, failing eyesight can minimize the fruitfulness of this possibility as a course of action. If an aid is purchased, a period of auditory training with the aid is necessary. The aid may prove beneficial under some circumstances but not others. If the aid never makes life more pleasant, it should not be worn.

The remainder of this section describes types of hearing loss, and the result of such loss, both to the person affected and to those who associate with him.

If the perception of all speech sounds depended solely on the fundamental frequency of laryngeally-vibrated tones, our hard-of-hearing problems would be significantly less than they actually are. Not all speech sounds are formed by vibration in the larynx. Many of our sounds are so-called *voiceless* sounds, i.e. they are created without vibration of the vocal folds. They are the result of turbulence of the air being forced through very narrow channels in the mouth or of the explosion of air after being momentarily stopped. The characteristic frequencies at which the sound power in these sounds is located are much higher than the fundamental frequencies of laryngeal tone. For example, whereas the fundamental frequencies for various vowel sounds produced by a man might range roughly from 125 to 150 Hz, the majority of the sound power in that same man's "s" sound will be concentrated above 4,000 Hz. In saying the word *saw*, the identifying characteristic energy concentration would move from frequencies above 4000 (for the "s") down to frequencies below 570 Hz (for the vowel sound [ɔ]).

If the auditor's hearing mechanism is unable to perceive frequencies above 5000 Hz at normal conversational levels but is able to perceive in the range of 125 to 2400 Hz, he will hear *awe*, not *saw*. Other voiceless sounds such as "t" and "th" (as in "thumb") require reception of frequencies above 4000 Hz in order to be heard. Similarly "f," "k," "sh," "p," and "ch" require high frequency perception if they are not to pose hearing uncertainties.

Certain other sounds such as "z," "v," "g," "zh," "dz," "d," and "b," include both the high frequency elements necessary for distinguishing them, in addition to the power concentration at the considerably lower frequency ranges due to laryngeal vibration.

In the flow of the spoken word, signals are sent out requiring receipt of rapidly fluctuating frequency and intensity levels. If the receiver is to be able to discriminate the sounds (and subsequently integrate them into meaningful units), his hearing *acuity* (ability to be aware of the presence of sound) must enable him to receive frequencies at least as high as 6,000 Hz. Hence, the hearing mechanism must be capable of successfully dealing with sounds over a fairly wide frequency range.

The certified audiologist learns a great deal about a case's hearing through administering a pure tone hearing test by means of an audiometer. He samples the case's acuity at discrete points along the frequency spectrum important to speech reception. He ascertains how much sound power is necessary to raise sounds of given frequencies above the threshold of hearing and hence elicit a response. These response levels are charted on a form called an audiogram. Testing is normally accomplished as 125, 250, 500, 1000, 2000, 4000, and 8000 Hz. The octave interval frequencies, appearing along the horizontal line, are plotted against the hearing level on the vertical line, in units of sound power called decibels (dB). Low pitches appear to the left and high to the right; faint sounds are represented at the top and loud at the bottom of the vertical line. When the levels achieved at each frequency are connected across the form with lines, the resultant *curve* yields a considerable amount of information about the person's hearing. Such air conduction thresholds are designated by a circle for the right ear and an "X" for the left. If a masking sound is delivered simultaneously to the nontested ear, the symbols △ and □ are used to represent right and left ears, respectively.

If the curve is *flat*, that is to say if most of the frequency range is depressed relatively equally (i.e. if there is a relatively equal threshold worsening across all frequencies), a *conductive loss* is suggested. Another way to say this is that if it takes X-amount of additional sound power throughout the frequency range in order for the person to perceive the presence of sound, he has a *conductive* type loss. Although flat sensorineural losses do occur occasionally, the flat loss is more often indicative of problems of the middle or outer ear — problems which frequently respond to professional intervention.

If more and more units of sound power (dB) are necessary to hear the successively higher frequency levels (i.e. the higher the frequency the higher the threshold rise), the resultant *falling curve* plotted on the audiogram indicates a *sensorineural loss.* The loss of acuity for the higher frequencies is usually an indication of an inner ear, and hence irreversible, problem.

If the audiologist's findings so suggest, further testing is done to compare the results of bone conduction audiometry (in which a vibrator is positioned behind the ear on the mastoid) with those

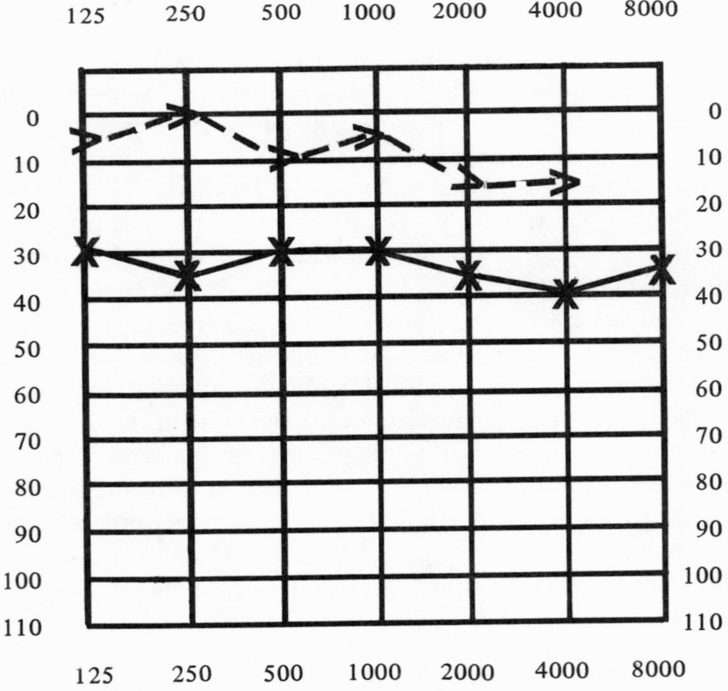

Figure 1. Audiogram showing conduction impairment (results shown for left ear only).

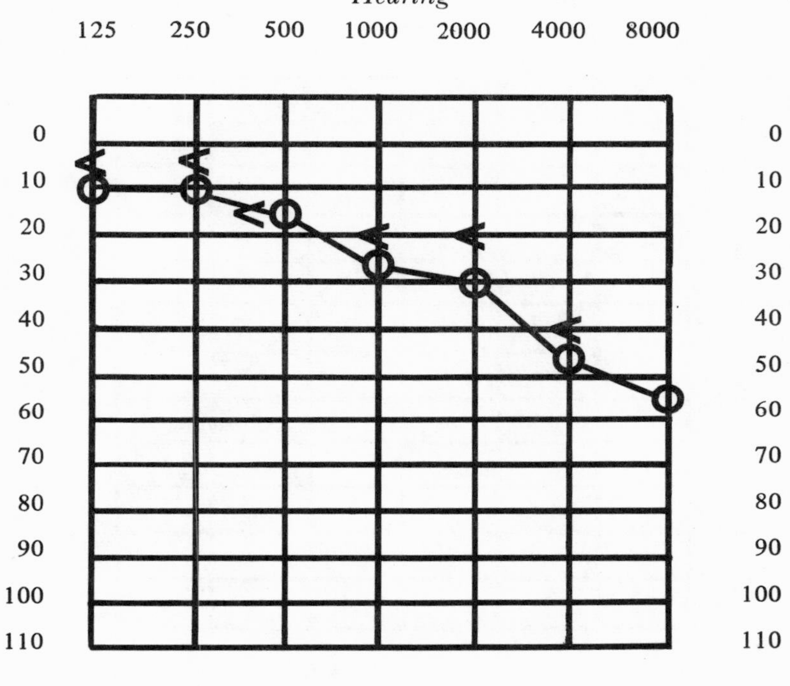

Figure 2. Audiogram showing sensorineural impairment (results shown for right ear only).

obtained through air conduction through earphones. The series of decibel levels indicated by bone conduction (BC) brackets (> for the right ear and < for the left ear) denotes the level at which the given Hertz values were heard by means of bone conduction testing. The symbols [and] are used if the opposite ear is *masked*. Examples of audiograms* illustrating the two main types of configurations are pictured in Figures 1 and 2.

In Figure 1 the *normal* contour of the bone conduction responses indicates no problem in the inner ear. The elevated threshold for the air conduction test indicates, in conjunction

---

*The illustrations given are basically grids with test frequencies represented on the abscissa (horizontal axis) and hearing level represented on the ordinate (vertical axis). Individual clinics specify the additional information to be included on the audiogram form.

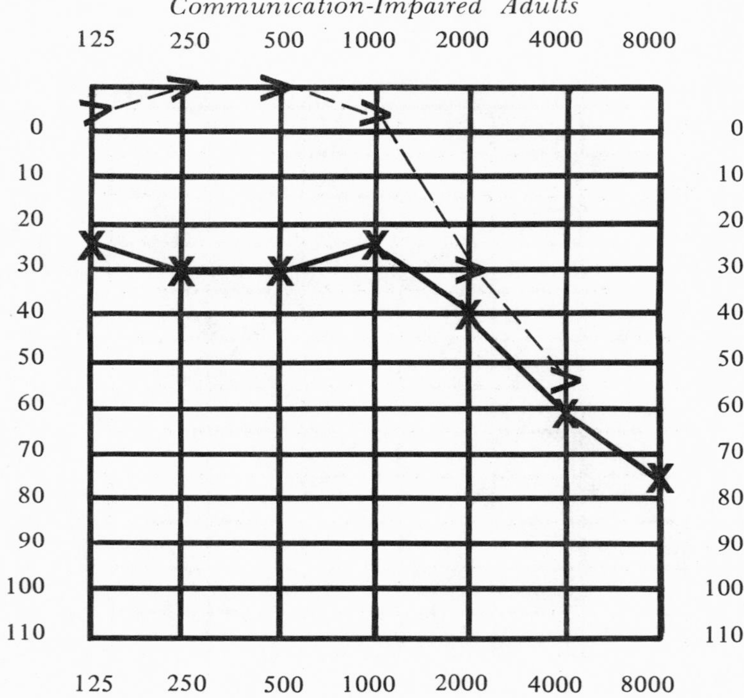

Figure 3. Audiogram showing mixed impairment (results shown for left ear only).

with the bone conduction information, that there is a conductive loss.

In Figure 2 a bone conduction curve following approximately that of the air conduction curve would indicate a sensorineural (formerly referred to as *perceptive*) loss.

The third main type of hearing loss configuration is a combination of the conductive and the sensorineural losses, as in Figure 3.

Were audiogram interpretations always as simple as delineated in these examples, the need for a large professional labor pool of audiologists would be considerably diminished. Unfortunately, hard-of-hearing persons seldom have such unequivocally easy audiograms to interpret. However, knowing this much about reading an audiogram will certainly help all of us to share our professional insights into given cases with a reasonable degree of clarity.

Often the audiologist must proceed to test via speech audiometry, in which standardized word lists are presented under both sound-field conditions (through loud speakers in an acoustically treated sound suite) as well as through earphones. By this and various other means, the audiologist ascertains the case's sound discrimination abilities. Speech audiometric techniques are indispensable in ascertaining the need for, or type of, hearing aid.

The human ear is not equally sensitive at all frequencies. Accordingly, a weighting system was built into standard audiometers to make all test frequencies equally loud at a level approximating the *normal threshold of hearing*. Reflecting more rigorous criteria, the 1964 standards of the International Organization for Standardization (ISO) supplanted the earlier (1951) American Standard Association's (ASA) standards. Tables are available depicting the decibel differences at each test frequency (e.g. p. 172 of the Rose-edited *Audiological Assessment)*. These have subsequently been replaced by American National Standard Specifications for Audiometers (ANSI) (see American National Standards Institute, Inc., 1970). Audiograms should indicate the given standards to which the audiometer utilized in testing was calibrated.

In summary, we can consider two main types of hearing problems arising out of impairments of the ear mechanism. In the one case — the conductive loss — if the power of the sound signal is increased sufficiently, the person can hear almost as well as before the loss. In the sensorineural loss, the higher frequencies may not respond to treatment. As the high frequency loss encroaches upon the frequency ranges necessary to the reception of speech sounds, these are *lost,* and the resultant verbal flow begins to sound like an irregular series of somewhat distorted vowel sounds separated either by *blurry* sounds, or by momentary silences. Perhaps of even greater importance than the loss itself is the attitude of the person who begins to react to a high frequency loss with disgust at "the slovenly speech of everyone these days." Nor does he appreciate being yelled at, since the increased loudness does not compensate for the absent high frequencies.

PRESBYCUSIS

In the process known as aging, the mechanism of the ear — like other parts of the anatomy — undergoes change. Elasticity and responsiveness are affected.

The very existence of the term *presbycusis* reflects the fact that everyone can expect to experience hearing difficulties if he lives long enough. It refers to the consequences of irreversible physiological changes of the hearing mechanisms. It is usually viewed as a sensorineural problem.* It typically begins after the age of fifty with gradual loss of acuity for the higher frequencies. The loss increases in severity and encroaches upon increasingly lower frequencies. Usually both ears are affected at approximately the same rate. The loss probably starts with changes in the ear mechanism itself (primarily inner ear) and progresses into the auditory nerve fibers, rises through the brain stem, and ultimately reaches the auditory areas of the cerebral cortex. Neither medical nor surgical treatment can significantly improve the presbycusic patient's hearing.

The chief complaint of the aging is not that they do not hear, but that they do not understand. *Phonemic regression* (Gaeth, 1948) may be reflected in a much poorer speech discrimination score than the pure tone audiometric findings would suggest. Difficulty in discrimination ability is usually experienced initially in noisy environments. The individual usually begins to seek help by the time he is having trouble understanding in quiet surroundings. The individual experiences particular difficulty in understanding rapid speech and in understanding speech while surrounded by other people conversing — either among themselves or seeking to gain his attention.

Additional factors that affect hearing include "noise, nutritional factors, psychological factors, and listening habits" (Barr, 1970). Glorig has used the term *sociocusis* to describe hearing losses due to noise conditions of our social environment,

---

*See Aram, Glorig and Hallowel, Davis: "Age, Noise and Hearing Loss. *Annals of Otology, Rhinology and Otolaryngology, 70*(2)556-71 (1961) for elaborations to, and exceptions from this generalization; and Harold F. Schuknecht, "Further Observations on the Pathology of Presbycusis," *Archives of Otolaryngology, 80*:369-82, (1964).

i.e. "those changes that may be ascribed to 'wear and tear' regardless of occupation" (Glorig, 1962). The frequent accompaniment of psychological difficulties increases the severity of the hearing problem. Acquired hearing loss is frequently associated with feelings of depression and isolation. This feeling of not being a part of things usually comes at a time when physical disabilities have already curtailed the individual's activities, and possibly resulted in withdrawal. The tendency for withdrawal, plus restriction of interests, adds to our difficulties in communicating with the elderly hard-of-hearing. Family members and associates, and hospital and nursing home personnel, need to understand the frightening aspects of such isolation.

The individual's physical and psychological condition poses problems for audiometric testing and assessing the possible benefits of a hearing aid. For high frequency hearing loss, it must be remembered that a hearing aid will probably do little to improve discrimination — it just amplifies. Since it amplifies *all* sounds in the environment, not just speech, the individual with an aid cannot tolerate it perpetually but will probably be more comfortable with it off in noisy environments. Hence the conscientious nurse's aide who strives to see that the individual *never* forgets his hearing aid, or who *never* forgets to turn it on, is providing a misguided and probably nondesired *service* to the patient or resident.

A hearing aid is not the ultimate answer for every hard-of-hearing person. Effective use of a hearing aid requires skill and insight. It depends on threshold sensitivity and discrimination ability, as well as life-style and motivation. Efficacy of speechreading assistance and auditory training also depends on motivation and life-style, as well as on time and money. Only the strongly motivated will gain from hearing aids and training.

THE USE AND CARE OF HEARING AIDS

For those persons who use an aid, there is the ongoing need to continually check the functioning of the instrument. As the hard-of-hearing individual ages, declining vision, arthritic fingers and arms, and encroaching senility affect his ability to check his own hearing aid. Hopefully the individual living with one or more family members can rely on those people to do the necessary checking if he is unable to do so. Patients in hospitals and residents in nursing homes and homes for the aged must depend on the nurse, nurse's aid, or other interested and *informed* personnel.

Typical complaints of aid users include the following:

1. Voices don't sound natural — they sound different, *tinny*.
2. My aid picks up more noise than speech.
3. I hear speech louder, but I can't understand it.
4. The aid makes a whistle-like sound.
5. I am bothered by the noise my clothing makes.
6. My aid does not seem to work right in extremely cold weather.

Hopefully the first three of these complaints should have been minimized through understanding gained during hearing aid orientation procedures at the time the aid is purchased. The fourth complaint suggests a defective instrument, loose earmold, or closeness of the microphone of a body type aid to the receiver. The fifth complaint can be met by putting the microphone on soft cotton or flannel clothing, not on synthetics or starched materials. The difficulty cited in the sixth complaint is probably temporary and should cease as soon as one's body temperature sufficiently warms the aid. These and many similar problems are normally anticipated and discussed during orientation sessions on how to use and care for an aid. For various reasons the aid user may be unable, or become unable, to satisfactorily solve the problems arising from aid usage.

Practical difficulties in the use of hearing aids arise from deterioration of vision, memory, and manual dexterity.

Visual problems impinge on the usefulness of aids when they render impossible the required setting of numbers, colored dots, or directional plus and minus signs. Poor vision can also prevent seeing if the mold is plugged and if the aid is corroded.

Failing memory introduces such problems as (1) forgetting which ear takes the aid; (2) forgetting to turn the aid off or on, as appropriate; (3) forgetting to change the battery; (4) getting old and new batteries mixed up (*always* throw out the old battery immediately upon changing); and (5) forgetting the right settings. (In hospitals and nursing homes this information should appear in the patient's medical chart).

Poor manual dexterity, particularly resulting from arthritic fingers and arms, can result in (1) problems in changing batteries; (2) failure to get the mold inserted properly in the ear; and (3) inability to work on-off and loudness controls.

Any listing of problems, such as the above, should make readily apparent the need of many hard-of-hearing persons to receive routine help from someone in their daily environment. Such assistance, if it keeps him satisfied, will probably be the major factor in keeping the patient in touch with society, preventing the retreat to isolation.

All aids, whether body type, ear level (including eyeglass aids), or all-in-ear, are *amplification* systems. As such, they are comprised of three main components in addition to a power source (battery): a microphone (which converts sound waves into an electrical equivalent of the acoustic signal), an amplifier and an earphone or receiver (which reconverts the amplified electrical signal into sound waves which are directed to the ear). Most aids have an on-off switch, a volume control (continuously adjustable or in steps, e.g. mild, moderate, or maximum gain), a battery compartment, a cord or tube, and an earmold. Other features, such as a telephone pickup and automatic volume control (to amplify sounds weak in energy such as "s") are incorporated to meet special hearing problems.

What are some of the basic checks that can be made by family members, nurses, aides, etc? The following series of checks might profitably furnish a basis for hospital and nursing home in-service training:

1. Is the aid operating? (Put the receiver — earphone — over the microphone, i.e. cup it in your hand. If the aid is working, it will whistle.)
2. Does the aid have a battery?
3. Is the battery the correct size and voltage?
4. Is the battery voltage good? (A battery tester will supply the answer. Average battery life is from 80 to 160 hours, dependent on

usage. Critical factors are how long the aid is worn daily and at how high a setting.)

5. Is the battery put in properly? (Some aids are designed so that the battery cannot be incorrectly inserted; others require lining up plusses and minuses on the battery with those on the aid to achieve the right polarity.)

6. Are dead batteries mixed with good ones?

7. Are batteries jostled with coins, keys, or any metal? ("Even a momentary 'short' can reduce the total operating battery life by many hours" (Berger and Millin, 1971).

8. Are contact points on both battery and case corroded? (A pencil eraser or an emory board can be used to clean the contact points.)

9. Are any foreign objects (such as food) stuck in the tubings, switches, openings, earmold? (Check the plastic tubing of an eyeglass or behind-the-ear aid for moisture blockage or for collapse of the tubing. It is wise to keep some spare tubing on hand.)

10. Is the microphone clean? (Food spillage can play havoc with a microphone.)

11. Is the earmold clean (free of wax, etc.)? (To clean, soak for a few minutes in mild soapy water, then scrub with a toothbrush. A pipe cleaner or toothpick can also prove helpful. Unless you are a doctor or nurse, do not clean the individual's ear!

12. Does the aid squeal when worn? (If so, is it broken? Does the ear mold fit properly? Is there breakage at any junction? Is the tubing cracked?)

13. Is the earmold tubing cracked? (Tubing should be replaced yearly.)

14. On large body aids is there a break in the wires? (Bend the wire back and forth while the aid is on to see if you get disruption. If so, it needs replacement.)

15. Is the cord inserted properly? (i.e. on aids with a telephone pickup, is the microphone [M] end erroneously inserted into the telephone [T] opening?)

16. Is the switch set to "M" for microphone and not "T" for telephone?

17. Is the aid set at the appropriate power setting?

18. Is the microphone opening covered over?

If none of these checks or suggestions improve the aid's performance, the aid should be seen by a manufacturer or experienced hearing aid technician to repair or replace the defective component. It might be profitable to ascertain whether or not hair sprays may have entered the microphone, whether water entered the microphone (if the patient bathed, showered, or washed his hair with the aid on), and whether or not the aid was dropped. Any of these activities could result in an aid's requiring factory servicing.

REFERENCES

American National Standards Institute, Inc.: *American National Standard Specifications for Audiometers (ANSI S3.6-1969),* New York, 1970.

Barr, David F.: Aural rehabilitation and the geriatric patient. *Geriatrics, 25(6)*:111, 1970.

Berger, Kenneth W., and Millin, Joseph P.: Hearing aids. In Rose, Darrell E. (Ed.): *Audiological Assessment.* Englewood Cliffs, P-H, 1971, Chap. 14.

Gaeth, John: *A Study of Phonemic Regression Associated with Hearing Loss.* Unpublished doctoral dissertation, Evanston, Northwestern University, 1948.

Glorig, Aram, and Nixon, James: Hearing loss as a function of age. *Laryngoscope, 72(11)*:1596, 1962.

Rose, Darrell E. (Ed.): *Audiological Assessment.* Englewood Cliffs, P-H, 1971.

Travis, Lee Edward (Ed.): *Handbook of Speech Pathology and Audiology.* New York, Appleton, 1971.

ADDITIONAL READING LIST

Alpiner, Jerome G.: Audiologic problems of the aged. *Geriatrics, 18(1)*:19, 1963.

Alpiner, Jerome: Diagnostic and rehabilitative aspects of geriatric audiology. *ASHA, 7(11)*:455, 1965.

Anonymous: Hearing loss in the aged. *Eye Ear Nose Throat Mon, 42(7)*:64, 1963.

Babbitt, James A.: Progressive deafness, otosclerosis and closely related subjects. *Laryngoscope, 50(5)*:385, 1940.

Bender, Ruth E.: Communicating with the deaf. *Am J Nurs, 66(4)*:757, 1966.

Bergman, Moe: Changes in hearing with age. *Gerontologist, 11(2)*:148, Summer, 1971, part I.

Bergman, Moe: Effects of aging on hearing. *Maico Audiological Library Series, Report 6,* 1967, vol. II.

Berkowitz, Alice O., and Hochbert, Irving: Self-assessment of hearing handicap in the aged. *Arch Otolaryngol, 93(1)*:25, 1971.

Bloomer, H. Harlan: Communication problems among aged county hospital patient. *Geriatrics, 15(4)*:291, 1960.

Calvert, Donald R.: Deaf voice quality: A preliminary investigation. *Volta Review, 64(7)*:402, 1962.

Campanelli, P. A.: Audiological perspectives on presbycusis. *Eye Ear Nose Throat Mon, 47(1)*:3, 1968.

Carhart, Raymond: The advantages and limitations of a hearing aid. *Minnesota Med, 50(6)*:823, 1967.

Carhart, Raymond, and Tillman, Tom W.: Interactio of competing speech signals with hearing loss. *Arch Otolaryngol, 91(3)*:273, 1970.

Davis, Hallowell, and Silverman, S. Richard: *Hearing and Deafness,* 3rd Ed., New York, HR&W, 1970.

Fibush, Esther W.: The problem of hearing loss. *Social Casework, 36(3)*:123, 1955.

Gaitz, Charles M., and Warshaw, H. E.: Obstacles encountered in correcting hearing loss in the elderly. *Geriatrics, 19(2)*:83, 1964.

Glorig, Aram: *Noise and Your Ear.* New York, Grune, 1958.

Goetzinger, C. P.: Management of hearing problems in persons of advanced age. *Eye Ear Nose Throat Mon, 42(1)*:38, 1963.

Goetzinger, C. P., *et al.:* A study of hearing in advanced age. *Arch Otolaryngol, 73(6)*:60, 1961.

Griffing, Terry S., and Hallberg, O. Erik: The audiogram and the hearing-aid problem in the aged. *Postgrad Med, 31(5)*:485, 1962.

Hardy, William G.: The hearing aid — for whom does it work? *Postgrad Med, 34(5)*: 436, 1963.

Harless, Edwin L., and Rupp, Ralph R.: Aural rehabilitation of the elderly. *J Speech Hear Disord, 37(2)*:267, 1972.

Hinchcliffe, Ronald: The anatomical locus of presbycusis. *J Speech Hear Disord, 27(4)*:301, 1962.

Hoople, Gordon D.: Care of hearing in the elderly. *Geriatrics, 15(2)*:106, 1960.

Hoops, H. R., and McLauchlin, R. M.: Reliability of conventional audiometry in the aphasic. *J Audiology Res, 9(3)*:240, 1969.

Hudson, Atwood: Communication barriers of the older person. *Ill Med J, 118(4)*:219, 1960.

Hunter, William F.:The psychologist works with the aged individual. *J Counsel Psychol, 7(2)*:120, 1960.

Jones, Wendell E.: Hearing loss in the aged. *Professional Nurs Home, 9(11)*:30, 1967.

Kirikae, Ichiro, Sato, Tsunemasa, and Shitara, Tetsuya: A study of hearing in advanced age. *Laryngoscope, 74(2)*:205, 1964.

Klotz, R. E., and Kilbane, Marjorie: Hearing in an aging population. *N Engl J Med, 266(6)*:277, 1962.

Kodman, Frank Jr.: Some attitudes of unsuccessful hearing aid users. *Eye Ear Nose Throat Mon, 40(5)*:405, 1961.

Kodman, Frank Jr., and Fine, Arthur: Some attitudes of successful hearing aid users. *Eye Ear Nose Throat Mon, 38(12)*:1027, 1959.

Kryter, Karl D.: The effects of noise on man. *J Speech Hear Disord Monograph Supplement I,* 1950.

Lehman, Roger H., and Miller, Alfred L.: Presbycusis. *Am Geriatr Soc J, 18(6)*:486, 1970.

Levine, Edna Simon: The psychological implications of hearing impairment. *Am J Occup Ther, 7(1)*:9, 1953.

Lindenberg, Paul: Deafness: Problems of diagnosis and rehabilitation. *Am J Occup Ther, 7(1)*:5, 1953.

Menzel, Otto J.: Psychological aspects of hearing impairment. *Eye Ear Nose Throat Mon, 42(8)*:72, 1963.

Miller, Maurice H.: Audiologic evaluation of aphasic patients. *J Speech Hear Disord, 25(4)*:333, 1960.

Miller, Maurice H.: Audiological rehabilitation of the geriatric patient. *Maico Audiological Library Series, Report 1,* 1967, vol. II.

Miller, Maurice H., and Ort, Ruth G.: Hearing problems in a home for the aged. *Acta Otolaryngol, 59*:33, 1965.

Minifie, Fred D., Hixon, Thomas J., and Williams, Frederick: *Normal Aspects of Speech, Hearing, and Language.* Englewood Cliffs, P-H, 1973.

Myklebust, Helmer R.: *The Psychology of Deafness,* 2nd ed. New York, Grune, 1964.

Newby, Hayes A.: *Audiology,* 3rd ed. New York, Appleton, 1972.

Olsen, Wayne O., and Tillman, Tom W.: Hearing aids and sensorineural hearing loss. *Ann Otol Rhinol Laryngol, 77(4)*:716, 1968.

Parker, Willard: Hearing and age. *Geriatrics 24(4)*:151, 1969.

Punch, Jerry L., and McConnell, Freeman: The speech discrimination function of elderly adults. *J Auditory Res, 9(2)*:159, 1969.

Ronnei, Eleanor C.: Hearing aids. *Am J Nurs, 63(5)*90, 1963.

Rosen, Samuel and Olin, Pekka: Hearing loss and coronary heart disease. *Arch Otolaryngol, 82(3)*:236, 1965.

Rosen, Samuel, *et al.*: Presbycusis study of a relatively noise-free population in the Sudan. *Ann Otol Rhinol Laryngol, 71*:727, 1962.

Rosenwasser, Harry: Otitic problems in the aged. *Geriatrics, 19(1)*:11, 1964.

Rupp, Ralph R.: A program of therapy-management for individuals with presbycusis. *Michigan Hearing, 19(2)*:5, 1969.

Rupp, Ralph R.: Understanding the problems of presbycusis: An overview on hearing loss associated with aging. *Geriatrics, 25(1)*:100, 1970.

Rupp, Ralph R., McLauchlin, Robert M., Harless, Edwin, and Mikulas, Marguerite: The specter of aging — golden years or tarnished. *Hearing and Speech News,* Nov-Dec, 1971, pp. 10-13.

Sataloff, Joseph, and Menduke, H.: Presbycusis. *Arch Otolaryngol, 66*:271, 1957.

Sataloff, Joseph, and Vassallo, Lawrence: Hard-of-hearing senior citizens and the physician. *Geriatrics, 21(12)*:182, 1966.

Schaie, K. Warner, Baltes, Paul, and Strother, Charles R.: A study of auditory sensitivity in advanced age. *J Gerontol, 19(4)*:453, 1964.

Schuknecht, Harold F.: Presbycusis. Laryngoscope, *65(6)*:402, 1955.

Schuknecht, Harold F., and Igarashi, Makoto: Pathology of slowly progressive sensori-neural deafness. *Trans Am Acad Ophthalmol Otolaryngol, 68*:222, 1964.

Scheer, Alan Austin: Rehabilitation of the hard of hearing. *Eye Ear Nose Throat Mon, 36(10)*:593, 1957.

Siegenthaler, Bruce M., and Gruber, Vera: Combining vision and audition for speech reception. *J Speech Hear Disord, 34(1)*:58, 1969.

Sklar, Maurice, and , and Edwards, Allan E.: Presbycusis: A factor analysis of hearing and psychological characteristics of men over 65 years old. *J Aud Res, 2(3)*:194, 1962.

Stone, Virginia: Hearing programs for our older population. *Nurs Outlook, 12(11)*:54, 1964.

Strong, E. C. Naylor: Deafness in the elderly. *Nurs Mirror, 129(2)*:19, 1969.

Upton, Hubert W.: Wearable eyeglass speechreading aid. *Am Ann Deaf, 113(2)*:222, 1968.

Weston, T. E. T.: Presbyacusis — a clinical study. *J Laryngol Otol, 78*:273, 1964.

Willeford, Jack A.: The geriatric patient. In Rose, Darrell E. (Ed.): Audiological Assessment. Englewood Cliffs, P-H, 1971, Chap. 9.

Winchester, Richard A., and Hartman, Bernard T.: Auditory dedifferentiation in the dysphasic. *J Speech Hear Disord, 20(2)*:178, 1955.

Chapter 5

STROKE

To the person fortunate enough not to have experienced a stroke in his immediate family circle, it is almost impossible to realize the enormity of the problems faced by the poststroke patient and members of his family. The problem of understanding these cases is further complicated by the wide variability of disabilities exhibited by any group of poststroke cases. These can include physical paralysis or pareses, sensory and perceptual decrements, intellectual changes, impaired memory span, impaired ability to concentrate, fatigability, increased irritability, uncontrollable emotional lability, and decreased interest in everyday activities. This chapter concentrates upon the poststroke individuals who manifest problems in communicating. It will deal in a subsidiary way with the frequently concomittant problems of paralysis. This book will bypass any discussion of so-called *little strokes,* but the reader interested in these phenomena will want to read the classic book by Dr. Alvarez on the subject (Alvarez, 1966).

Perhaps the scope of the problem is best and most succinctly stated by Arthur C. Jones. In *Care of the Patient with a Stroke,* Jones observes that "Loss of voluntary control of any part of the body is a disturbing event. Loss of control of all of one side of the body is a disaster. Loss of the ability to communicate is a catastrophe" (Smith, 1967).

Unfortunately for the poststroke victim, our society seems ill-equipped to tolerate the loss of the use of a part of the body, impairment of mental activity, or speech incapacities. From active participation in work, church, community affairs, and leisure time pursuits, the patient can become almost completely inactive and estranged from family, peers, and friends. The stroke patient's family is most worried about whether he will continue to be crippled — either motorically or in speech. The family members are most apt to ask "Will he talk again?" "How long will it take for him to talk again?" "Will he go back to work?" "How soon can he return to work?" "If he is left with permanent disability, what are his chances for returning to work — be it his present job, or another?"

THE FIRST POSTSTROKE MONTHS

In view of the problems presented, it is necessary that patient care plans include a series of goals such as self-care, independent ambulation, reentry into comfortable group relationships, and resumption of community roles. As important as communication is in achieving these goals, most speech pathologists do not immediately commence direct speech restorative techniques. Of higher immediate priority than verbal communication are such matters as the ability to recognize one's mate, interest in personal grooming, self-respect, fatigue levels, visual problems, appropriate nutrition, concerns about sex, epileptic control (if involved), depression, suicidal tendencies.

Prior to initiating either language diagnostic procedures or direct therapy, it has been customary until fairly recently for speech pathologists to delay their services until major spontaneous recovery had been achieved — usually within three to four months postonset. By this time, it was assumed that the euphoric phase would have passed, that emotional lability would no longer be evident, and that language behavior would have reached a plateau (Wepman and Jones, 1967). Such delay might also be related to the reduced reliability of prognoses made prior to the achievement of neurological stability.

However, it is during this period of so-called *spontaneous recovery* that both patient and members of his family are in greatest need of counseling and guidance from any and all of the rehabilitation personnel, be they therapist, social worker, psychologist, physician, etc. While attempting to cope with the multitudinous problems involved, it is frequently with the nurse that the patient first tries to talk and with whom he first discovers his frightful language disability. It is during this period that members of the patient's family must be heard; they need to complain, to minimize, or rid themselves of their anxieties.

The earliest management of the hemiplegic patient himself is equated with good rehabilitation nursing care, i.e. the nurse must "relinquish her desire to do everything for the patient and to stop thinking of the patient as a passive recipient" (Jennings, 1967). The nurse either reinforces the patient's desire for self-care and independence, or she smothers it. Above all other specialists, the nurse must proceed from early intensive care to a supportive, yet demanding, role.

The management of emotional factors is as crucial as the prevention of contractures, decubitus ulcers, and urinary tract infections — all of which can complicate recovery if prolonged bedrest is involved. Reassurance and support are crucial needs. The primary roles of acute hospitals are to save life and to make the patient medically stable. Since the stroke case tends to become physically stable relatively quickly, he is frequently sent to nursing homes rather than being held in rehabilitation wards of acute hospitals.

It might be well for everyone involved in poststroke care to heed the advice proffered by Leonard D. Policoff in the March, 1970, edition of *Geriatrics*. His article on "The Philosophy of Stroke Rehabilitation" concludes as follows:

> The rehabilitation of the stroke patient represents, in microcosm, the fundamental philosophy of rehabilitation medicine — to ensure comprehensive medical diagnosis and management, to cope with the environmental and psychosocial aspects of disease and disability as strenuously as with their pathological aspects, to provide ongoing supervision and follow-up care as long as the patient's condition requires it, and to utilize the resources of a team of physicians and allied health professionals working with common, coordinated purpose and objectives to achieve the maximum functional restoration of the individual, even when the basic pathology or its residua cannot be corrected. The salvage of individuals from the nursing-home scrapheap more than justifies the effort" (Policoff, 1970).

Of greatest importance for immediate care is the ability to chew and swallow, the ability of the patient to make his wants known, the ability to use "yes" and "no" responses, and the ability to follow verbal commands without visual clues. The extent of impairment (if any) of these abilities and the resultant implications must be interpreted to the patient's family and to the staff involved. A major challenge to all concerned is how to avoid the patient's "retreat to the 'wisdom' of silence" (Dr. Basilio Lopez, 1971, in addressing a class of graduate speech pathology students). Patients anticipating lifelong debilitation tend to exhibit withdrawal characteristics secondary to the brain damage.

The physician's and nurse's interest in good nutrition for the case is usually attributable to different factors than those of interest to the speech pathologist. While the nurse's problems are fewer if intravenous feeding can be avoided, the speech pathologist is even more directly interested in the patient's ability to chew and swallow, i.e. activities which require action of the speech muscles. To the nurse, diets are chiefly a means of meeting bodily needs for sustenance or for controlling certain health problems such as diabetes; for the speech pathologist they are crucially related to use of the speech musculature.

The speech musculature must not be allowed to atrophy through disuse. It is of crucial concern to the speech pathologist that *someone* — be it nurse, nurse's aide, dietitian, occupational therapist, or speech pathologist — teach sucking, swallowing, and chewing techniques if there is muscular impairment. The presence of drooling should always stimulate further examination of the ability to suck, chew, and swallow. Drooling, when sitting up, suggests facial/oral paralysis. In reflecting upon medical mistakes, Dr. Milton M. Hurwitz, in describing the remarkable recovery of a so-called *hopeless stroke* case, concluded "It seems likely that more vigorous attempts to try to get the patient to regain some ability to swallow should have been made much earlier" (Hurwitz, 1970).

The speech pathologist's interest in patient alertness is shared equally by other members of the staff. We are all interested in the patient's ability to utilize auditory, visual, tactile, and emotional inputs. If one makes better contact by standing on one side of the patient or the other, we should suspect the visual problem known as homonymous hemianopsia. If the patient is hallucinating, and is presenting *confused* speech, it might be best to delay speech and language therapy. Language behaviors common to most aphasics include greatly diminished vocabulary size (the most severe cases may be limited to automatic or emotional speech), a reduced verbal retention span, grammatic (sentence structure) and semantic (word meaning) confusions, varying degrees of ability to comprehend spoken and written words, and writing problems.

Not all communication impairments are attributable to the stroke. The patient may have visual or auditory problems that preceded the stroke. Did he possess glasses or hearing aids? Are the glasses and hearing aids available to him in the hospital or nursing home? Has the patient's vision been further impaired by the brain damage?

Dentures, too, can play a part in the patient's speech difficulties. The author recalls one case referred to speech pathology as an *aphasic*. A gentleman in his late seventies had suffered a stroke. The hospital personnel having contact with him could not understand him — hence referral to the speech pathology service. Shortly after meeting and listening to the patient, the speech pathologist asked the patient to remove his dentures and to speak up, saying she was hard-of-hearing. Whereupon, the miracle of speech was restored. (The dentures were so ill-fitting that the patient had to continually hold up the uppers with his tongue to prevent them from falling. The resultant speech distortion, along with a basically weak voice, rendered his speech unintelligible to the rest of the staff.) While this case greatly increased the prestige of the speech pathologist, perhaps other staff members should have been more alert. Perhaps the diagnosis of *aphasia* could have been avoided.

While the patient is still in bed, the speech pathologist's initial assessment is concerned with the patient's ability to follow simple directions, to respond appropriately to questions requiring *yes* or *no* answers, and to express himself. Can he make speech sounds? Is his speech slurred? Does he have word-finding difficulties? Can he read? Can he write? The disabilities encountered dictate the nature of the speech pathologist's staff recommendations and family counseling. A foreign language background can add to the problems of verbal expression.

The speech pathologist's concern during the immediate poststroke period is with the patient's most basic needs. Similarly the nurse, the nurse's aide, the physical therapist, and the occupational therapist are interested in activities of daily living. These specialists can do their work more effectively if they work hand-in-hand with the speech pathologist on basic need words and short commands (which may need to be augmented with standardized gestures, or pictures, dependent upon the severity of the patient's language problems).

A lot of old wive's tales have arisen, plus some major problems, over the imprecision of the professional literature on when speech pathology services should begin. Dependent upon which writings the given physician may have been exposed to, he may tend to withhold speech pathology referrals until three months (or six) have elapsed. Still others, noting the passage of six months' time, while they have followed through on a drug regimen augmented by physical therapy, will observe that spontaneous recovery is now complete and little good can come of further rehabilitation efforts. Still other physicians, having waited for the patient's poststroke depression to recede, make referrals one, two, and even three years poststroke.

On the other hand, some physicians refer cases almost immediately poststroke to speech pathologists who may, with a given case, participate in bedside chewing, sucking, and swallowing assistance to restore activities necessary for speech and language production.

What implications do these various poststroke delays have for the speech pathologist's work? Certainly they affect greatly his choice of diagnostic tools. Obviously his chance to use differing evaluative techniques depends greatly upon the philosophy and rapport of the various specialists involved in the rehabilitation team of which he is a part.

The very presence or absence of a speech pathology referral effectively extends or limits the speech pathologist's services. How many left hemiplegics, for example, have been discharged from the hospital without the speech pathologist ever knowing of the case's presence in an acute ward? The brevity of the attending physician's attention to his speech, and the patient's frequent verbosity, often are judged to preclude a needed speech pathology referral. However, who else will discover his impaired auditory memory span, impairment of his arithmetic processes, his difficulties in time and space? In many cases it is the speech pathologist who uncovers this cluster of problems which certainly should be considered in the discharge plans — in planning continuity of case care.

At the opposite referral extreme is the referral for "intensive vocabulary retrieval" for the case with such severe oral paralysis that direct speech and language techniques *at that time* would actually be contraindicated.

Rather than setting an arbitrary number of poststroke days or weeks for initiating speech pathology evaluation, many pathologists now do preliminary examinations and initiate treatment procedures as soon as the patient begins to relate to his environment and can sit up for two hours without fatigue. This timing can be as variable as the patients themselves are variable in both their prestroke and poststroke behaviors. Schuell concluded that "it still seems wise to withhold differential diagnosis and prognosis for recovery from aphasia until patients are neurologically stable. This statement does not imply that treatment should necessarily be deferred until this time, however" (Schuell and Nagae, 1969).

One of the gravest errors one can make is to look at poststroke cases as *stereotypes*. It is extremely necessary for everyone involved to share with each other their insights into the individual patient and his family environment. Frederick Greenberg sums up quite well the speech pathologist's early role in the patient's recovery by stating "An attempt is made... to provide the rehabilitation team, referring physician, and patient's family with descriptive information on the patient's language, so that those in his environment can best communicate with him" (Peterson and Olsen, 1965).

Perhaps the timing of initial speech pathology referrals will shortly resolve itself as more and more rehabilitation centers adopt the Porch Index of Communicative Ability (PICA) as a primary speech diagnostic/prognostic tool. At present, the accuracy of prognosis based on PICA findings depends greatly upon using this test instrument *exactly one month* postonset. Increased acquaintance of physicians with the values derived by the speech pathologist's use of this test should help greatly in minimizing the problems attendant upon severely delayed speech pathology referrals.

RECENT APHASIA DIAGNOSTIC TESTS

The nonspeech pathologist, upon discovering the many aphasia diagnostic tests available, might have cause to question the reasons for such proliferation. Perhaps the number simply reflects the continuing search for better ways to understand and to treat individuals who exhibit diverse kinds of language impairment. The enormity of this search is reflected in Hildred Schuell's conclusion that "an adequate diagnostic test must sample relevant kinds of behavior in all language modalities over the entire range of aphasic deficit" (Schuell, 1972). As Wepman and Jones noted "there is no panacea, no single special method, no time-proven technique that explains aphasia or that always succeeds in its treatment. The challenge is just as great today as it was about 30 years ago when the condition turned from being a symptom in neurological diagnosis to its present status as a therapeutic problem" (Wepman and Jones, 1967)

The survey of aphasia diagnostic tests appearing in Appendix B is limited to a description of tests published within the past dozen or so years, with capsule comments on advantages and possible disadvantages of their use. No attempt will be made to delineate all of the background considerations of test construction. Instead, a pragmatic look is taken at the reasons for testing and the relationship of these needs to the characteristics of the given tests. After initial identification, each of these tests subsequently will be referred to by the initials appearing in parentheses after the test name.

While it might seem expedient to select diagnostic tests on the basis of cost, durability, ease of administration, proficiency in classifying patients, or time required to administer, score, and analyze, many speech clinicians are likely to consider other criteria more important for test selection. They are probably most interested in what the patient can or cannot do at that point in time, since such information on language ability and disability will provide guidelines for treatment. This purpose appears to many clinical aphasiologists to be of greater importance than diagnosing, in the sense of *categorizing* the patient — fitting him into a given system of classification. They are interested in test and tester reliability in order to document confidently therapy progress as well as to compare test results with scores obtained on the same test administered by different clinicians. They are interested in tests which yield a dependable prognosis.

They may be interested also in the arrangement of items on a given test — for example, tests in which the individual tasks appear in order of decreasing ability, thus leaving the patient with feelings of success at the end of the testing. They may be more interested in functional than in clinical (specific-task test-situation) skills. In any event, they need to evaluate the effects of any impairment of perceptual and motor skills upon language performance in all modalities. They need to differentiate aphasia from dysaghria, oral apraxia, apraxia of speech, mental deterioration, and/or emotional problems.

The speech and language clinician's choice of tests is further influenced by the severity of the patient's communication breakdowns, as well as by whether the concomitant paralysis is right- or left-sided. The choice of tests can also be influenced by their appropriateness to purposes other than patient care — for example, for research, teaching, counseling, and helping to determine site of lesion.

APHASIA TERMINOLOGY

Diagnostic and therapeutic techniques leading to better patient care have been changing rapidly in the past decade. Accordingly, it would seem prudent for health and allied health professionals to proceed cautiously in responding to nonqualified diagnostic labels attached to poststroke cases who demonstrate communication difficulties. The team approach to patient care — so widely pursued in rehabilitation settings — should do much to obviate inept and inappropriate custodial and treatment procedures. Total comprehensive care is a necessity, with each of the various specialists communicating with each other about the patient.

Any assumptions that all poststroke cases demonstrating communication problems are *aphasia* are quickly dispelled in the case staffings of such teams of specialists. As more poststroke cases enter nursing homes and homes for the aged, the challenge to render the best possible services extends wider and wider. Nurses and their aides can derive greater satisfactions from their work as they come to better understand the diverse problems of those entrusted to their care.

There is probably no other disorder treated by rehabilitation specialists in which there is such extensive and confusing terminology in use as is the case with aphasia. This is due to the fact that it has been classified in terms of anatomy, linguistics, physiology, and psychology, dependent on the bias and background of the classifier. A systematic analysis of all classifications of aphasia would constitute by itself a separate, large volume. However, one need not react with discouragement or a sense of futility to this situation. A few major distinctions are mandatory and can be clearly delineated. Additional terminology to be mastered by any given allied health specialist will probably depend upon the training and preference of the speech pathologist involved and of the physician heading the department or institution in which he works.

Perhaps the initial matter to clarify is the use of the prefixes *a-* and *dys-*. There are spokesmen for the view that use of the prefix *a-* connotes a complete lack of, while use of the prefix *dys-* indicates a partial lack or impairment of (something). The incidence of varying degrees of severity of language impairment versus complete impairment of language abilities would suggest that if one term were to evolve, it probably should be *dysphasia*. However, common usage does not always appear to follow the most logical pattern of development. In the recorded history of centrally-impaired language problems, the word *aphasia* has been used so widely to refer to all degrees of impairment — even the most minimal — that present insistence on a meaningful distinction from *dysphasia* seems somewhat absurd. This book recognizes the peculiar historical development of the labeling of language impairments due to brain damage by treating the words *aphasia* and *dysphasia* as if they were synonymous.

Of far greater importance, particularly because of ihpliiatit s for treatment, is the necessity to distinguish any of the aphasias from dysarthria, oral apraxia, and apraxia of speech, sometimes referred to as verbal apraxia. (Note: the preceding list reflects the prefix usage which seems to be currently preferred with these several diagnostic labels.)

There are many definitions in existence for the term *aphasia*. Most such definitions include two main concepts: (1) impaired ability to interpret and formulate language symbols, and (2) causality — i.e. brain damage — "disproportionate to impairment of other intellective functions; not attributable to dementia, sensory loss, or motor dysfunction" (Darley, 1969). The impaired abilities include word finding problems (slowed vocabulary retrieval), syntactic errors (inappropriate grammatical constructions or lack of grammatical completeness), semantic errors (inappropriate meaning), reduced auditory retention span, problems in understanding or comprehending what is heard, and problems in reading and writing language and/or arithmetic symbols.

Dysarthria (sometimes called *anarthria*) is a speech (or motor deficiency), rather than a language (symbolic) problem. Its basis is some type of abnormality of the central or peripheral nervous system controlling the speech mechanism. Dysarthria refers to "problems in oral communication due to paralysis, weakness, or incoordination of the speech musculature" (Darley, Aronson, and Brown, 1969). Dysarthria manifests itself in distortions and substitutions of speech sounds. Distortion is consistent; hence, speech sound errors tend to be predictable. The sound distortion is frequently accompanied by monotonous voice quality, labored rate, and in some cases, by hypernasality. The Mayo Clinic group (Darley, *et al.*, 1969) appear to have either clarified or expanded the term *dysarthria* "to encompass coexisting motor disorders of respiration, phonation, articulation, resonance, and prosody (those variations in time, pitch, and loudness which summate to produce emphasis and interest in speech)" Darley, *et al.,* 1969).

In the broadest sense an agnosia is a loss of the function of recognition — an inability to recognize the import of sensory stimuli due to brain damage. A visual agnosia could involve form, size, color, letters, numbers, words. An auditory agnosia could involve sounds, words, and/or music. Inability to recognize objects by feel (tactile) is called *astereognosis.*

An *apraxia* — sometimes referred to as a *sensorimotor disorder* — is an inability to perform skilled purposeful acts through loss of memory (due to brain damage) of how to perform them. Aphasia is frequently accompanied by various agnosic (receptive) and apraxic (expressive) elements.

According to Darley, *apraxia of speech* — sometimes referred to as *Broca's aphasia* — is "an articulatory disorder resulting from impairment, as a result of brain damage, of the capacity to program the positioning of speech musculature and the sequencing of muscle movements for the volitional production of phonemes. The speech musculature does not show significant weakness, slowness, or incoordination when used for reflex and automatic acts" (Darley, 1969). Articulation errors are inconsistent and usually occur on the consonant sounds beginning words. These errors include substitution of one consonant sound for another, repetition of sounds, addition of sounds, and sound omissions.

The verbal apractic's errors are highly variable, unlike the consistency of the dysarthric's errors. There is a deterioration of articulation with increasing length of words or phrases and with increased word *weight*). Apraxic subjects usually are aware of their errors. There is noticeable groping or struggle-like behavior with repeated attempts. The articulation tends to improve on several consecutive attempts to produce the desired response.

In *oral apraxia* — not to be confused with *verbal apraxia* — patients display "difficulty in responding to commands to protrude their tongue, pucker their lips, blow, chatter their teeth, whistle, etc." (Johns and Darley, 1970).

Assisted with at least these few diagnostic distinctions, let us proceed to a closer look at the problems faced by poststroke individuals and their families.

FAMILY COUNSELING

McKenzie Buck, a professor of speech pathology who fought his way back from severe poststroke aphasia, notes that "a stroke is actually a family illness and continuous counseling should be readily available for the entire household" (Buck, 1964). He feels that professional personnel are obligated to provide regular and lengthy opportunities for nondirective family counseling. In a talk presented during the summer of 1958, Dr. Buck stated that "under no circumstances will I ever again initiate any therapy with this type of patient without being convinced that the family has enough objective information to evaluate the sick member and understand his reactions."

Among some of the first questions asked by family members faced with a stroke are "What happened?" and "Why did this happen?" The first question is far easier to answer and to understand than the second. If the stroke was vascular (pertaining to blood vessels) in origin, it should be relatively easy for the attending physician (or nurse or medical social worker) to explain the necessity for the brain to be furnished oxygen by means of the bloodstream. Anything that disrupts the flow of blood to the brain for more than three or four minutes can cause irreparable harm.

The major vascular disturbances are embolism, thrombosis, hemorrhage, mechanical occlusion, or vasospasm. An *embolism* is the sudden plugging of a blood vessel by a blood clot or by a foreign body (dead cell tissue) borne by the bloodstream to its present location. The obstruction is called an embolus. A *thrombosis* is the formation, by coagulation of the blood, of a plug or clot which remains at the point of its formation and results in the slow occlusion of a vessel by thickening its wall or lining. This stationary obstruction is called a thrombus. A *hemorrhage* is an abundant escape of blood due to rupture of a vessel, leading to extravasation of blood into the surrounding tissues. This results in both a toxic effect upon the area getting the spilled blood, as well as a deprivation to the area which would have been furnished the blood. *Mechanical occlusion* is brought about by pressure from without the vessel due to a neoplasm (any new and abnormal growth such as a tumor). A *vasospasm* is a temporary narrowing of the vessel under the influence of hormones or vasoconstrictor nerves.

The attending physician may be able to cite the specific type of vascular condition at fault, or he may be prepared to discuss with the family other possible etiologies including infectious processes, degenerative brain diseases, or allergic cerebral edema (presence of abnormally large amounts of fluid in the brain).

Discussion of why a given stroke happened might at first glance appear to have little benefit. However, even though it is impossible to return to the patient's premorbid condition by taking steps to counteract hypertension, high blood cholesterol levels, heart disease, inadequate exercise and rest, obesity, cigarette smoking, and diabetes (factors considered to increase the likelihood of stroke), the family must be made to realize that recurrence of a stroke is most likely if the risk factors which resulted in the stroke are not significantly alleviated or eliminated.

The family must also be brought to understand that there are no medicines, drugs, or surgery known which can *cure* the poststroke condition. However, there are medications which can help the patient's physical or emotional conditions.

The family must further be brought to understand that the condition is neither *catching* nor progressive, although it is apt to appear worse at times (probably due to fatigue, depression, and emotional stress). Nor is the condition a sign of mental incompetency.

The family members definitely must be taught to expect changes in personality and general behavior. For example, poststroke cases tend to fatigue more easily, they have shorter attention spans, they demonstrate less interest in people and hobbies, they are more irritable, they have difficulty remembering recent events, they may be confused about time and place, they have a greater tendency to laugh and cry, and a greater ability to get upset over seemingly little things. Some patients may lose all interest in personal tidiness or appearance (or, conversely, become overly concerned with cleanliness). They may give way to physical violence. If the family is not apprised of these possibilities, they will assuredly suffer even more in their attempts to cope with such unexpected conditions.

The family may need counseling on the handling of convulsive seizures. Of particular importance is the prevention of seizures. McKenzie Buck (1968, p. 39) supplies a helpful list of behavioral deviations which would suggest the need for neurological reevaluation of the patient. These are:

1. Sudden attacks of extreme fatigue.
2. Frequent demonstrations of spontaneous hyperirritability, sometimes accompanied by self-punishing behavior.
3. Periodic increases in verbal and behavioral confusion.
4. Instantaneous disruptions in verbal expression.
5. Unexplained pains in any part of the body, particularly when these occur in the paralyzed side that has not previously demonstrated a sensory response.
6. Attacks of extreme stomach upset resulting in vomiting.
7. Agitated restlessness for no apparent reason.
8. Excessively severe headaches.
9. Lightning flashes in the visual field (Buck, 1968).

It is imperative that the patient be kept in a language environment. He should not be shunned because he appears not to comprehend. When talking with the patient, it is necessary to be relaxed — not in a hurry. If a person is unavoidably rushed, and yet must talk with the patient it is best to word all questions in a form that demands only *yes-no* responses.

It is the extent of the family member's knowledge and insight into the patient's problems (and how to deal with them), and his ability to maintain favorable attitudes, that will most affect the patient's progress. The family must maintain cheerfulness with the patient and give him both emotional support and reassurance, as well as the motivation to continue to work on his problems. Each professional involved needs to maintain a positive outlook. He must be realistic about expectations for progress without conveying pessimism.

Underlying all the family's efforts must be an adequate approach to at least three basic living needs. Since a characteristic of brain damaged individuals tends to be excessive fatigue (which serves to enhance failure), it is imperative that the patient get adequate *physiological rest*. The usual combination of decreased vitality with reduced emotional and intellectual controls bodes ill for recovery.

A second basic need is adequate *nutrition*. One must beware of letting food become a solace for emotional distress, or a mere habit reaction to frustration. The third basic need is acceptable toiletry. While this word is used in its widest sense, to include personal grooming as well as voiding activities, the episode described by Buck (1968) on page 31 of his book should surely be brought to the attention of everyone associated in any way with stroke victims. Anyone reading about the relationship of reduced memory and physical mobility ending in incontinence will never forget Buck's message.

The literature on aphasia is almost barren of information on how the patient's family is affected by his condition. In an investigation of family members, via the interview technique, Russell L. Malone reports the following problems: role change, irritability, guilt feelings, altered social life, financial problems, job neglect, health problems (due to disturbed rest), over-solicitousness, and rejection (Malone, 1969). These attitudes suggest the need for intensive counseling in order that the family members might become positive members of the rehabilitation team. They must understand what the patient's limitations are, how they will affect him, and how this will affect their relationship to him.

The family members should realize, too, that the patient, like themselves, is undoubtedly worried about everything, not just language loss alone. If the patient is severely depressed there may be suicide attempts. Dr. Buck, having unsuccessfully tried to commit suicide himself, suggests that the family see to it that kitchen knives and razors (nonelectric) are not readily available. He suggests that family members keep an eye on the patient since loneliness can lead to suicidal depression. This is particularly a problem when the wife works all day and the children are at school. Dr. Buck asks whether the wife can take employment where the patient can accompany her, such as in a nursing home or restaurant.

Dr. Louis B. Newman notes that "a stroke paralyzes the persons around the patient, too. We must train the family of the patient in their new roles, so that they can learn to handle their own anxiety at the patient's condition, and to help the patient achieve independence rather than lapse into confirmed and permanent disability" (Newman, 1966) Dr. Buck amplifies this type of caution, indicating the real possibility of an overprotective family hindering the patient's progress. He prides himself on his obstinacy in insisting on putting on his own raincoat, without help from his wife. A sign of Dr. Buck's considerable recovery was, as he narrates, when he began to feel sorry for the people hanging around who wanted to help him, and decided to let them help.

The family needs to educate the neighborhood, as well as close friends, about the patient's emotional outbursts. The patient needs *the heat taken off*. It is easy for family members to quickly forget their own prestroke ignorance about aphasia.

One must continously remind himself that most people know nothing about aphasia. Most people talk too fast for the aphasic to understand, and frequently they shout in order to make themselves understood. Everyone needs reminders to not shout, to speak slowly and clearly, to get his attention before speaking and then speak directly to him and to speak in short — but not childish — sentences. At no time should the patient's capacity to understand be underestimated.

The potential improvement of the patient's functional ability is closely related to the family's understanding, particularly their nonverbal behaviors which enable the patient to perceive their total response to his problem. The patient needs to feel needed and wanted by his family. He must have tasks to perform, responsibilities to assume. Because his wife may need to become the major breadwinner of the family, the patient may have difficulty accepting a lesser *provider* role than prior to his stroke. Yet progress will depend on the skill of the patient and his spouse in readjusting to different role demands.

Immediate poststroke family questioning will quickly move into the area of prognosis. Prognosis seems to be a highly individual matter, although prognosis for physical rehabilitation obviously is directly related to such residual involvements as the following, enumerated by Mieczyslaw Peszczynski: bowel incontinence, urinary incontinence, knee flexion contractures, sensory involvement, pain, motivation, special problems arising from multiple lesions, upper extremity involvement, and gait (Peszczynski, 1963). Although his article concentrated on factors involved in *physical* recovery, Peszczynski added that the rehabilitation potential of the late adult hemiplegic further depends upon a sympathetic environment if he is to be able to utilize his remaining capabilities.

Other factors which have been advanced as potentially playing an important role in recovery include age (the younger the better), etiology (trauma-incurred aphasics have a greater recovery hope than vascular-incurred), personality (extroverts tend to do better than introverts), and earliness of the initiation of speech and language training (the earlier the better). Additional factors are educational or occupational level; the extent of injury to brain tissue; the degree and type of communication disorder; presence of related perceptual, sensorimotor, or dysarthric components; whether or not the pathology is progressive; the general medical stability of the patient; the patient's environment, including economic pressures and degree and type of family stimulation; whether or not the patient had been using his intellectual powers for further learning; the patient's physiological, intellectual, and social maturation; his motivation; his emotional stability; his awareness of error and ability to correct himself; and the skill of each member of the rehabilitation team.

All rehabilitation specialists can be of greatest assistance if they achieve a well-rounded picture of the patient's prestroke environment and life-style. Whether this information is gathered by a medical social worker, by a nurse, an aide, a psychologist, or by the speech pathologist, a good pretraumatic history gathered by the appropriate personnel is a must. It is necessary to know how the patient lived and worked. Of specific concern is the patient's interests; hobbies; occupation; work patterns; educational level; probable intellectual level; personality; presence of significant auditory, visual, or dental problems; his family (including their attitudes and insights); etc.

Presuming an at least minimally cooperative family constellation, the appropriate family members should participate in the various therapy sessions. This is particularly necessary in that the patient forgets, making for little follow through of therapeutic activities. And the patient gets blamed for not doing what he forgot! It might be appropriate to indicate here that in a nursing home, the aide serves as the family.

In the presence of no speech, or isolated words only, some families have labeled almost every article in the home. These labels are pointed out while repeating the word again and again. For this severe a case, speech pathologists usually welcome similar help from all the professionals involved (PT, OT, nurse, etc.) in repeated repetition of the names of commonly used words. It is of the utmost importance to the patient to regain words like toilet, comb, lipstick, razor, eat, water, sleep. If vocabulary retrieval is going to involve such strenuous effort, let us be sure that we all concentrate on the most needed words!

Attention should be called to the added problems attendant upon discharge to the patient's home. The patient is forced to cope with role changes within his family at the very time that the present health care and social service systems desert him. A laudatory project in the author's home community trains volunteers to enter the home of a hospital-discharged poststroke patient and assist him and members of his family to "maintain or further develop his maximal potential within a life-style acceptable to him and his family and community" (Mayer and Scott, 1972).

A number of publications intended primarily for the families of poststroke individuals are available. A selected list of these appears in Appendix C.

LEFT HEMIPLEGIA

While poststroke communication problems can occur without paralysis, the frequency of these problems occurring together is so great that we will discuss two main poststroke types — aphasia accompanied by right-sided paralysis (i.e. left hemisphere cortical involvement), and left hemiplegics (individuals with paralysis of the left side of the body whose behavioral changes are associated with damage to the right cortical hemisphere).

Thus far most of our discussion of poststroke problems applied equally to individuals suffering either right or left hemisphere damage. However, the comments made about *language* thus far pertain primarily to the person with right-sided paralysis. This section attempts to delineate problems frequently accompanying left hemiplegia. It should be understood that these problems are *likely* to be encountered within this population, but by no means should *all* of these problems be expected in every patient whose left side is paralyzed.

Disturbances of body image, spatial judgment, sensory interpretation, and visuomotor skills are significantly limiting factors affecting poststroke progress. Also, the left hemiplegic "finds innumerable excuses to avoid treatment, fails to keep his appointments, antagonizes the staff, and does little to assist his rehabilitation" (Knapp, 1966). Accordingly, left hemiplegics tend to be known as *difficult* patients, and generally have a poor prognosis for independent functioning. A quick comparison of the right hemiplegic and the left hemiplegic is afforded by juxtaposing the speech findings for the two ennumerated by Dr. Miland E. Knapp (1966). His listing of impairments is as shown in Table II.

The left hemiplegic, quoting Dr. Knapp, "seems to lose some inhibitory factor, talks too much but does not use good judgment in what he says and does not follow up his words with actions. He may insist repeatedly that he is anxious to work hard to get well, but stops working after only minimal effort" (Knapp, 1962).

Although the left hemiplegic's world may not have changed significantly, his perception of it is almost invariably changed. Perception is defined by Burt (1970) as "the ability to integrate and interpret all the sensory messages from our internal and external environment. This ability is the result of the combined activity of the end organs, peripheral nerves, tracts and ganglia, and the integrative sensory cortex" (Burt, 1970). The left hemiplegic's difficulty in monitoring time stems from a shortened attention span. For example, he may forget whether or not he took his medicine. Such forgetfulness can impair medical treatment if he fails to use his medication. On the other hand, overdosage can produce different complications. Similarly, a rapid spurt in body weight might suggest forgetfulness with

Table II

Speech Findings: Left Hemiplegia	*Speech Findings: Right Hemiplegia*
Impaired integration and judgment	Impaired recognition
Impaired time concepts	Impaired retention
Impaired spatial concepts	Impaired recall
Impaired drawing, writing, and body assembly	Dysarthric qualities
Impaired written mathematics	Impaired abstract language
Impaired reading comprehension	Impaired comprehension
Errors are inconsistent and patient is usually not aware of them	
There is no apparent mental damage because they are able to express themselves well, but careful examination shows some very serious defects concerning the visuomotor, temporal, and spatial concepts, particularly in the judgment and abstract generalizations related to these concepts. These defects may cause more difficulty than lack of speech in rehabilitation.	The casual observer usually gets the impression that the patient is mentally damaged because his speech is poor... However, mentation is generally good in spite of a severe speech difficulty.

From Miland E. Knapp, "Lecture 2. The Hemiplegic Patient — Rehabilitation," *Postgraduate Medicine, 39(3)*:A-143 (1966).

respect to eating. Because he cannot remember that he ate, he eats again. And again. And again!

Although he may be able to *read* the clock, he may be unable to monitor time intervals. He is confused over the amount of time that has elapsed since last performing a given action. This can have dire effects on his eating, medication, exercise, and other regimens. His complaints about getting no lunch, or of treatments being skipped, can cause all kinds of havoc in the relationships of family and staff members who may be unaware of this problem.

His time confusion might reveal itself in his discussion of things supposedly done recently. He may accurately narrate a morning's activities that were routine before the illness, as if they were actions he had just experienced. For example, in discussing *this* morning's activities, he may discuss driving down to the marina, scraping and varnishing parts of his boat, taking a sail, jogging over to the club for a cup of coffee, and driving back home in time for lunch. Yet in actuality he has been confined to a wheelchair all morning in his hospital room.

He experiences many problems as the result of spatial neglect and distortions of spatial judgments. For example, he may find himself unable to complete the task of dressing. He may dress only one side of his body. He may get into his clothes backwards or upside down, attempting to put his feet and legs into his sweater sleeves, and attempting to get his arms into his trouser legs. He may get into his trousers and get angry with the fool that sewed up his fly — not recognizing that he put his pants on backwards and that the fly with its zipper is presently in back.

He may ignore or deny the left side of his body. He might give either of his two paralyzed limbs a name, such as "Johnnie," "Mack," or "the Sick One." Similarly, upon being asked to draw a man, he might draw only half of a body — the right side of a person.

Whether due to ignoring, denial, loss of tactile awareness of the left half of his body, or simply the inability to see things or activities past the midline toward the involved side, he may shave only the right side of his face, comb the hair on the right side of his head, eat from the right side of his tray or place setting, write only on the right side of a book (or read only the right side of a page), etc. He will frequently fail to accommodate the left side of his body when going through doors — while attempting to walk, or while attempting to manipulate his wheelchair. Such walking attempts end up in bruises; such wheelchair efforts can result in spinning the chair in circles. In preparation for leaving his wheelchair he may lock the brake and raise the footpedal on the uninvolved side, but forget to do the same on the involved side. He appears to require around-the-clock reinforcement on focusing to the left.

It should be noted that a visual field loss on the right frequently accompanies right hemiplegia. However, such field losses are not encountered as frequently as those accompanying left hemiplegia. In addition, the right hemiplegics tend to be far more amenable to treatment for visual field loss.

Because the left hemiplegic has difficulty localizing objects in space, he experiences difficulty in finding his way around his room. When leaving home or hospital he almost instantly becomes lost, unable to find his way back — even though he may be only next door or across the street! Since the left hemiplegic seldom finds his way back once lost, many nursing homes have put alarms on all doors to alert the staff when someone leaves the building. Obviously a person with these problems is a poor candidate for discharge to his own home unless he will have constant family supervision or live-in help on a twenty-four hour basis.

The left hemiplegic may experience letter reversals in reading and writing (e.g. "You light a fire with a *W*atch" and "You tell time with a *M*atch"). He might be able to read a paragraph aloud but be unable to comprehend its meaning. He may reverse his digits in attempting to work out written arithmetic problems, yet does not experience such problems in oral arithmetic. He may have difficulty in making change although retaining his ability to identify each coin in terms of its name and value. He may be unable to correctly write a check — not only from the standpoint of the value involved, but in terms of putting the date, the payee, and his own signature in the appropriate places. He may also be unable to dial a phone number successfully.

Again and again he demonstrates poor judgment. For example, although wheelchair-bound, he may proceed to get up to try to walk down the hall. He may forget to brake his wheelchair or lift up the footpedals when necessary. He may even attempt to descend a flight of stairs in his wheelchair.

He may be able to describe completely and explicitly a process or sequence of related events, yet be unable to follow through the sequence himself. For example, he may get out nails, hammer, and saw and then promptly forget what he was going to do with them. The left hemiplegic housewife might start assembling and combining the ingredients of a recipe, have her attention diverted to something else midway in the process, and completely forget to finish her cake. This can be especially aggravating when she forgets that something is cooking or baking.

Adding to the frustrations of those caring for the left hemiplegic is his apparent unawareness of his own errors and his frequent inability to recognize errors when pointed out to him.

Despite having one or more (or all) of the above-cited problems, it is possible for the left hemiplegic to comply satisfactorily with the various demands of physical examination and thus not be referred for a speech pathology examination. This is particularly true if the patient evidences no oral paralysis or its frequently concomitant dysarthria. This is possible because the left hemiplegic is generally free from normal aphasic involvement and would accordingly appear to have retained a high level of comprehension and expression. Some of the left hemiplegics actually talk incessantly — regardless of whether or not they had high pretrauma verbal output. However, Jon Eisenson observed that what is present in their speech is (1) "an increase in the number of words the individual needed to express his ideas," (2) "a looseness of verbalization," and (3) "more circumlocution (more hunting for the right word)" (Eisenson, 1962). Most physicians have not been trained to recognize such subtle communication differences.

A frequent complaint of speech pathologists employed in acute hospitals is that "We don't get left hemiplegic referrals because their speech is good." Neither are such referrals routine in rehabilitation hospitals, or rehabilitation wards, until the speech pathologist can demonstrate their need and values to the referring physicians.

Left Hemiplegia — Management

In attempting to cope with the problem of neglect of the affected side, the nurse can either arrange the patient's environment so that all vital objects (such as call light, nightstand) and activities are on the uninvolved side, or she can attempt to train the patient to attend to happenings on the involved side. The first option, while it might simplify life for the nurse, does little to assist the patient to regain independence. In following the second course of action, instructions must be given repeatedly — almost constantly. The reminder to "turn your head" must be given again and again and again. Food trays can be equipped with some type of brilliant stimulus on the left edge, the patients being continually instructed to turn until he can see it, thus allowing him to see all the food on the tray.

This same principle (to assist in focusing to the left) can be applied to dressing, reading, writing, and walking activities.

It is wise for everyone to approach the patient with a visual field cut from the patient's nonaffected side. This principle should be considered with respect to placement of his bed or his favorite chair in relation to the room's door and the room's center of activity. The entire staff and family must understand that success in self-accomodating to the left is rarely totally achieved. It must also be understood that this failure to turn is not the result of willful obstinacy. It is a condition, highly resistant to change, and hence highly frustrating to everyone involved in the patient's care. The therapeutic *hope* is that time and repeated effort will increase self-awareness of the neglected side.

Dressing can be facilitated by the use of color coding, e.g. color-coded markers can be used to indicate various aspects of the garment — front or back, left or right, top or bottom. Similarly, color coding can be used to facilitate joining objects such as the correct end of the electric cord with one's razor or other appropriate household appliances.

A full-length mirror may be of help to the patient experiencing distortions of the horizontal or vertical plane. It may help to achieve good sitting or standing balance. Timers, hourglasses, and radio and TV programs can be utilized in attempting to restore the ability to judge the passage of time.

Instructions must be carefully planned for brevity, simplicity of vocabulary and sentence structure, and singularity of command. Each command should consist of only one concept, i.e. the patient should not be told to take his medicine until he has complied with the preceding command to "sit up." Failure to wait until the first command is accomplished before giving the second may result in the patient's choking as he attempts to swallow the medicine while lying on his back. Hence, "Sit up and take your medicine" is a poor type of command to give a left hemiplegic. Directions must be in short, single-concept sentences, spoken slowly and clearly (yet not overexaggerated), and repeated if necessary. The primary essentials in all attempts to help the left hemiplegic are repetition, routine, and consistency.

Speech therapy for left hemiplegics begins with attempting to discriminate a correct from an incorrect response. Any reading, writing, or arithmetic retraining attempts must focus on getting the patient to compensate for his visual loss or neglect (if present). Improvement in judgment might be accomplished through role playing techniques including analysis of the characters' actions and decisions. Generally speaking, prognosis for left hemiplegics is *guarded* because most such individuals seem unable to learn from their mistakes.

Speech pathologists, at present, do a lot of improvising in testing left hemiplegics. No standardized diagnostic test has yet been constructed — to the author's knowledge — to deal satisfactorily with the majority of such patients. However, as long ago as 1958, Virginia Carroll isolated parts of the Schuell test which were helpful in detecting visuospatial impairment in left hemiplegic patients (Carroll, 1958).

COMMUNICATION OF THE APHASIC

This chapter is intended to be a practical help for the various people who interrelate with aphasics on a day-to-day basis, such as family members, nurses, and therapists. It is not intended as instruction in techniques for the speech pathologist. Hence, few of the articles on techniques used by speech pathologists appear in the chapter References and Additional Reading List. Such a purpose is not consistent with the philosophy of this book. However, many of the case handling suggestions contained herein are undoubtedly in use by speech pathologists.

It is most helpful to understand the various types of communication impairment demonstrated by the patient, or, conversely, the various communication skills remaining intact. Normally it is assumed that an evaluation of communication skills and deficits would be made by a speech pathologist and shared with all pertinent personnel.

The steps taken by a speechpathologist prior to initiating therapy are succinctly delineated by Edward J Lorenze and

Martin Sokoloff as follows:

> When an aphasic patient is referred to a speech clinic, a complete battery of tests is administered to determine the exact nature of his difficulties. On the basis of the results of these tests, an individualized program of language retraining is planned for him. Often this program involves not only re-establishing his vocabulary with word associations but also guiding him through the several levels of language functioning. The therapist observes the level at which language performance breaks down in the different modalities, determines critical dimensions of impairment within the individual modalities, evaluates the nature of the disturbances in language behavior, and identifies recurrent patterns of such disturbances. Then he sets goals for therapy and formulates a prognosis" (Lorenze and Sokoloff, 1967).

Initial and ongoing evaluation also includes observation of symbolic, personality and intellectual changes, memory, attention span, ability to abstract, and other behavioral characteristics.

If a speech pathologist's evaluation is unobtainable, assessment based on daily observations can be accomplished by any number of people concerned for the patient. Such a type of assessment is facilitated by the Wisconsin Division of Health's *Communication Status Chart* (Wis. Div. of Health, 1966). Similar assessment is discussed by Sidney Goda (Goda, 1963).

Anyone working with aphasics must recognize the tendencies of many aphasics for perseveration and catastrophic reactions. Demands must be reduced; task substitution is advisable. Warning signs of psychological breakdown are perseveration (meaningless repetition of a just completed and appropriate act), disinterest, excessive eye-blinking, irritability, and sweating.

Distinction between dysarthria (impairment of intelligibility) and aphasia (language impairment) is essential. The impaired articulation of the dysarthric can range from speech which is severely unintelligible to speech which is mildly unintelligible. Such extremes of *speech* production, concomitant with adequate *language,* can result in the listener's comprehension varying from total unintelligibility to single word intelligibility, through understanding short phrases, to understanding sentences with slight difficulty.

Aphasic disturbances involve impairment of symbolic processes both from the standpoint of reception (listening and reading) to speaking (including gestures and facial expressions) and writing.

Sidney Goda (1963) discusses levels of auditory verbal involvement — levels of understanding the heard word (usually evaluated in terms of response to directions and commands of varying levels of complexity) and levels of visual verbal involvement (different degrees of skill in reading). Similar levels of skill (or impairment) could be advanced with respect to writing. Besides introducing the reader to the complexity of communication involvements, Dr. Goda advances a number of excellent suggestions for understanding and helping the aphasic/dysarthric patient. He also notes the need to adapt to higher levels of language usage as growth in these abilities is noted in the patient.

As with the hard-of-hearing, the patient's speech efforts should be accepted. Patients must not be caused to feel shame for what they cannot do; they must be rewarded for what they can do. They must be encouraged to try to speak despite fear and frustration. One must attempt to communicate with aphasics at their own particular level of language functioning, even if it means learning the patient's gestural system.

It is easier to observe a patient's lack of speech than it is to recognize auditory problems of communicative significance. A potentially useful rule of thumb might be to assume difficulty in all areas of language — namely, auditory discrimination, auditory comprehension, auditory retention, verbal formulation and production, reading and writing. Therapists who are alert to sensory or perceptual deficits will structure their assistance so that the patient can deal most effectively with his total problem.

Another basic guideline is to be sure that the patient's attention is obtained before speaking. Then one should speak directly to the patient, clearly and slowly, yet maintaining normal phrasing and intonation. Sufficient response time must be allowed. One will be most successful if he uses simple sentence structure — keeping his comments and requests brief, simple, and containing one idea at a time. For example, commands can be given in single words, such as *watch, wait, listen,* and *swallow*. In attempting to serve their patients more adequately the writers of several patient care manuals on hemiplegia have rewritten their manuals, utilizing single commands in teaching transfer activities to people with short attention spans. (See the 1970 editions of the Wisconsin State Division of Health's pamphlets listed in this chapter's Additional Reading List.)

Talking louder or *talking down* are seldom appropriate. One may need to compensate for decreased auditory retention by frequently repeating, by repeating key words in sentences, by rewording the same thought, by using appropriate gestures to reinforce the spoken word. The patient may need to be prepared for shifts in conversation. The simultaneous use of visual and auditory stimuli is frequently appropriate.

Rehabilitation workers are encouraged to assist with what Hackworth and Best term "Language Activities of Daily Living, or L.A.D.L." (Hackworth and Best, 1965).

Wendell E. Jones and Charles H. Kramer offer good suggestions to nurses for understanding aphasic patients and for counseling the hospital staff and the patient's family (Jones and Kramer, 1967).

It is essential that all environmental persons — hospital or nursing home staff, as well as family members — understand the language of the patient and the goals and objectives of the rehabilitation efforts.

It is probably with aphasic patients that nursing and speech pathology can gain the most in understanding each other's professional activities and problems. For example, it is far more natural for a nurse to *do for them* than to *elicit speech from them*. If the nurse does not understand the value of encouraging her aphasic patient to speak, he may remain mute on the ward, even though he may be becoming talkative in the speech service. Even worse, the patient might interiorize that "They don't want me to try because they think I can't." Needless to say, such rationalization can only impede the aphasic's progress in communicating.

The meaning of an aphasic's inappropriate crying or laughing is also seldom understood by the patient's family and by other professionals. If the nurse takes these outbursts for granted, not responding to them, she is in a position to similarly advise the patient's family and friends.

The frequent use of profanity is also profoundly disturbing to the patient's family. His wife, sisters, and daughters cannot tolerate it — they do not know what to tell their neighbors. The aphasic patient is feared because of his inability to speak. The family must be counseled again and again (as well as the nursing staff).

Another nursing pitfall is to treat the aphasic patient like a child because he appears childlike, being unable to ask for his needs, constantly repeating, etc. It must always be remembered that his comprehension, alertness, and coherence *can be intact!* The staff must learn not to respond for the hesitant communicator.

The speech pathologist, in the absence of scientific support for the infallibility of any specific therapy approach, must select therapeutic procedures which seem appropriate for the given patient — approaches lying somewhere between the extremes of unrealistic pressures for language development and the dangers of having the patient become accustomed to a nonspeaking or poor response state. He will not only use specific stimulation approaches, but he will also incorporate nonspecific stimulation involved in sympathetic and encouraging environment, in concern for the patient's interests, hobbies, etc., in socialization approaches with other aphasics. He will attempt to capitalize upon the modality by which the given patient seems to learn most rapidly.

Although each member of the therapeutic team might contribute in his own way to the speech improvement of poststroke cases, they must be equally alert to the danger signs of undue frustration due to speech efforts and be able to tactfully ease out of communicative demands when negative results are obvious. To minimize well-motivated but undesirable language activities, one should maintain an active relationship with the speech pathologist involved in the case. The speech pathologist should be able to consult on which practices appear desirable and to what degree, as well as on which practices seem contraindicated. Ultimately, the family constellation of greatest benefit to the patient will almost intuitively begin to make the appropriate choices in their language interactions with the patient.

Opinions on the value of group therapy for aphasics are diverse. Apparently, much is thought to depend upon the type of individual therapy used concomitantly by the speech pathologist. The author of this book feels that if controlled behavioral modification techniques are impossible on an intensive basis, it seems fortuitous to utilize whatever resources are available, and these can include the directed use of group therapy, if only for as brief a time as a coffee hour. By assembling several aphasics for such a function and requiring some type of communication of everyone, the average aphasic usually experiences emotional support, encouragement, and motivation to continue work. He benefits from identification with others of similar circumstances; he finds understanding listeners.

Among the various specialists who express concern to see some rehabilitative speech work done with the patient who would not receive any therapy otherwise, is Barbara E. Miller, a nurse. She cites simple evaluative techniques in her article "Assisting Aphasic Patients with Speech Rehabilitation" (Miller, 1969) as well as therapeutic approaches. She remains mindful, also, of the patient's emotional, social, and motivational needs. It would appear that Ms. Miller's ideas might be best implemented as supplemental work done under the direction of a speech pathologist. While many might argue that few nurses would have the time to devote to these activities, Ms. Miller herself states that "There is no reason why the nurse cannot take an active part in speech rehabilitation for the patient with aphasia who would otherwise have no rehabilitation" (Miller, 1969).

REFERENCES

Alvarez, Walter Clement: *Little Strokes*. Philadelphia, Lippincott, 1966.
Buck, McKenzie: Adjustments during recovery from stroke. *Am J Nurs,*

64(10);92, 1964.

Buck, McKenzie: *Dysphasia: Professional Guidance for Family and Patient.* Englewood Cliffs, P-H, 1968.

Burt, Margaret M.: Perceptual deficits in hemiplegia. *Am J Nurs, 70(5)*:1026, 1970.

Carroll, Virginia: Implications of measured visuospacial impairment in a group of left hemiplegic patients. *Arch Phys Med Rehabil, 39*:11, 1958.

Darley, Frederic L.: Expressive Speech-Language Disorders. Partial transcript of presentation at American Speech and Hearing Association Convention, 1969.

Darley, Frederic L., Aronson, Arnold E., and Brown, Joe R.: Differential diagnostic patterns of dysarthria. *J Speech Hear Res, 12(2)*:246, 1969.

Eisenson, Jon: Language and intellectual modifications associated with right cerebral damage. *Lang Speech, 5*:49, 1962.

Goda, Sidney: Communicating with the aphasic or dysarthric patient. *Am J Nurs, 63(7)*:80, 1963.

Hackworth, Howard Bing, and Best, Jean: Practical therapy for aphasics. *Rehabil Rec, 6(5)*:19, 1965.

Hurwitz, Milton M. (Ed.): In retrospect — a look back at medical mistakes: "Hopeless" strokes. *Geriatrics, 25(1)*:48, 1970.

Jennings, Carol R.: The stroke patient — his rehabilitation. *Am J Nurs, 67(1)*:118, 1967.

Johns, Donnell, F., and Darley, Frederic L.: Phonemic variability in apraxia of speech. *J Speech Hear Res, 13(3)*:556, 1970.

Jones, Wendell E., and Kramer, Charles H.: Creating a therapeutic language atmosphere. *Professional Nurs Home, 9(9)*:46, 1967.

Knapp, Miland E.: Lecture 2. The hemiplegic patient — rehabilitation. *Postgrad Med, 39(3)*:A-143, 1966.

Knapp, Miland E.: Results of language tests of patients with hemiplegia. *Arch Phys Med Rehabil, 43(7)*:317, 1962.

Lorenze, Edward J., and Sokoloff, Martin: Management of aphasia. *Stroke, 2(1, 2)*: 1967.

Malone, Russell L.: Expressed attitudes of families of aphasics. *J Speech Hear Disord, 34(2)*:146, 1969.

Mayer, Hanno, and Scott, Antoinette: *Volunteers for Stroke: A Plan to Utilize Volunteers as Part of the Stroke Team.* Milwaukee, Sacred Heart Rehabilitation Hospital, 1972.

Miller, Barbara E.: Assisting aphasic patients with speech rehabilitation. *Am J Nurs, 69(5)*:983, 1969.

Newman, Louis B.: Forefront. *Geriatrics, 21(9)*:69, 1966.

Peszczynski, Mieczyslaw: The rehabilitation potential of the late adult hemiplegic.*Am J Nurs, 63(4)*:111, 1963.

Peterson, Jean C., and Olsen, Ann P.: *Language Problems After a Stroke: A Guide for Communication.* Minneapolis, Kenny Rehabilitation Institute, 1965.

Policoff, Leonard D.: The philosophy of stroke rehabilitation. *Geriatrics, 25(3)*:99, 1970.

Schuell, Hildred M.: A re-evaluation of the short examination for aphasia. In Sarno, Martha Taylor (Ed.): *Aphasia — Selected Readings.* New York, Appleton, 1972.

Schuell, Hildred, and Nagae, Kazuhisa: Stroke: U.S. and Japan — Aphasia studies. *Geriatrics, 24(10)*:141, 1969.

Smith, Genevieve Waples: *Care of the Patient with a Stroke: A Handbook for the Patient's Family and Nurse.* New York, Springer Pub, 1967.

Wepman, Joseph M., and Jones, Lyle V.: Aphasia — diagnostic description and therapy. In Fields, William S., and Spencer, William A. (Eds.): *Stroke Rehabilitation: Basic Concepts and Research Trends,* St. Louis, Green, 1967.

Wisconsin Division of Health (Section of Patient Care Practices): Communication Status Chart (Screening Test), Wisconsin Division of Health, 1966.

ADDITIONAL READING LIST

Aphasia — General

Agranowitz, Aleen, and McKeown, Milfred Riddle: *Aphasia Handbook for Adults and Children.* Springfield, Thomas, 1964.

American Heart Association: *Aphasia and the Family.* New York, American Heart Association, 1969.

Anderson, Thomas P., Bourestom, Norman, and Greenberg, Frederick R.: *Rehabilitation Predictors in Completed Stroke.* Minneapolis, Kenny Rehabilitation Institute, 1970.

Arffa, Marvin S.: Stroke patients in nursing homes. *Rehabil Rec, 9(2)*:30, 1968.

Baker, A.B., and Katsuki, Shibanosuke: Stroke: U.S. and Japan — Summary and conclusions. *Geriatrics, 24(11)*:124, 1969.

Benton, A. L.: Problems of test construction in the field of aphasia. *Cortex, 3(1)*:32-58, 1967.

Biorn-Hansen, Vera: Social and emotional aspects of aphasia. *J Speech Hear Disord, 22(1)*:53, 1957.

Bonkowski, Robert J.: Verbal and extraverbal components of language as related to lateralized brain damage. *J Speech Hear Res, 10(3)*:558, 1967.

Boone, Daniel R.: A plan for rehabilitation of aphasic patients. *Arch Phys Med Rehabil, 48(8)*:410, 1967.

Boone, Daniel R.: *An Adult Has Aphasia.* Danville, Interstate, 1965.

Brookshire, Robert H.: *An Introduction to Aphasia.* Minneapolis, BRK Publishers, 1973.

Brown, Jason W.: *Aphasia, Apraxia and Agnosia: Clinical and Theoretical Aspects.* Springfield, Thomas, 1972.

Buck, McKenzie: Dysphasia: The patient, his family, and the nurse. *Cardiovasc Nurs, 6(5)*:51, 1970.

Buck, McKenzie: Life with a stroke. *Crippled Child, 35(4)*:4, 1957.

Buck, McKenzie: The language disorders. *J Rehabil, 29(6)*:37, 1963.

Chen, Li-Ching Yen: "Talking hand" for aphasic stroke patients. *Geriatrics, 34(4)*:145, 1968.

Cohen, Lillian Kay: *Communication Problems After a Stroke.* Minneapolis, Kenny Rehabilitation Institute, 1971.

Corbin, Marria Lennon: Group speech therapy for motor aphasia and dysarthria. *J Speech Hear Disord, 16(1)*:21, 1951.

Culton, Gerald L.: Spontaneous recovery from aphasia. *J Speech Hear Res, 12(4)*:825, 1969.

Darley, Frederic L.: Impairment of communication ability in patients with cerebrovascular accidents. *Mayo Clin Proc, 42(10)*:648, 1967.

Darley, Frederic L.: Speech problems in the aging. *Postgrad Med, 33(3)*:294, 1963.

deReuck, A. V. S., and O'Connor, Maeve (Eds.): *Disorders of Language.* Boston, Little, 1963.

Derman, Sheila, and Manaster, Albert: Family counseling with relatives of aphasic patients at Schwab Rehabilitation Hospital. *ASHA, 9(5)*:175, 1967.

Eagleson, Hodge M. Jr., Vaughn, Gwenyth R., and Knudson, Alvin, B. C.: Hand signals for dysphasia. *Arch Phys Med Rehabil, 51(2)*:111, 1970.

Eisenson, Jon: *Adult Aphasis — Assessment and Treatment.* New York, Appleton, 1973.

Fawcus, Margaret: Group therapy for the aphasic patient. *Speech Pathol Ther, 7(1)*:30, 1964.

Fields, William, and Spencer, William A.: *Stroke Rehabilitation: Basic Concepts and Research Trends.* St. Louis, Green, 1967.

Fox, Madeline J.: Talking with patients who can't answer. *Am J Nurs, 71(6)*:1146, 1971.

Geschwind, Norman: Language and the brain. *Sci Am, 226(4)*:76, 1972.

Goldstein, Hyman, and Hamilton, Cameron: New method of communication for the aphasic patient. *Ariz Med, 9(8)*:17, 1952.

Goodkin, Robert: A procedure for training spouses to improve functional speech of aphasic patients. *Proceedings of the 77th Annual Convention of the American Psychological Association, 4 (Part 2)*:765, 1969.

Grey, Howard A.: The aphasic patient — and how you can help him. *RN, 33(7)*:46, 1970.

Griffith, Valerie Eaton: *A Stroke in the Family: A Manual of Home Therapy.* New York, Dell, 1970.

Hagen, Anton C.: Communication disorders of the stroke patient. *Clin Orthoped, 63*:102, 1969.

Halpern, Harvey: *Adult Aphasia.* Indianapolis, Bobbs, 1972.

Holland, Audrey L.: Case studies in aphasia rehabilitation using programmed instruction. *J Speech Hear Disord, 35(4)*:377, 1970.

Horwitz, Betty: An open letter to the family of an adult patient with aphasia. *Rehabil Lit, 23(5)*:141, 1962.

Houchin, Thomas Douglas, and DeLano, Phyllis Janes: *How to Help Adults with Aphasia.* Washington, D.C., *Pub Aff Pr,* 1964.

Hudson, A.: The rehabilitation team and the aphasic patient. *Am Arch Rehabil Ther, 20(2)*:58, 1972.

Johnson, Barbara: "Cook book therapy" for the aphasic. *Rehabil Rec, 8(2)*:20, 1967.

Jones, Juliet: The dysphasic patient in the neurosurgical department. *Speech Pathol Therapy, 7(2)*:78, 1964.

Jones Wendell E.: Working with the adult aphasic patient. *Professional Nurs Home, 9(10)*:32, 1967.

Keenan, Joseph S., and Brassell, Esther G.: A study of factors related to prognosis for individual aphasic patients. *J Speech Hear Disord, 39(3)*:257, 1974.

Keith, Robert L.: *Speech and Language Rehabilitation: A Workbook for the Neurologically Impaired.* Danville, Interstate, 1972.

Kottke, Frederic J.: Rehabilitation by specialists. *Rehabil Rec, 6(1)*:31, 1965.

LaPointe, Leonard L., and Culton, Gerald L.: Visual-spatial neglect subsequent to brain injury. *J Speech Hear Disord, 34(1)*:82, 1969.

Longerich, Mary Coates: *Manual for the Aphasic Patient.* New York, Macmillan, 1958.

Longerich, Mary Coates, and Bordeaux, Jean: *Aphasia Therapeutics.* New York, Macmillan, 1954.

Malone, Russell L., Ptacek, Paul H., and Malone, Marqueritte S.: Attitudes expressed by families of aphasics. *Br J Disord Commun, 5(2)*:174, 1970.

Marks, Morton, Taylor, Martha, and Rusk, Howard A.: Rehabilitation of the aphasic patient — a survey of three years' experience in a rehabilitation setting. *Neurology, 7(12)*:837, 1957.

Massengill, Raymond Jr., and Levinson, Carole: Management of the stroke patient with aphasia. *NC Med J, 28(6)*:233, 1967.

Micklish, Rita: Stiles, Anna E. (Room 201, Stroke). *Nurs Outlook, 14(11)*:44, 1966.

Mitchell, Joyce: Communication in the geriatric unit 3. *Nurs Times, 65(16)*:495, 1969.

Mitchell, Joyce: Disorders of communication in the older patient. *Gerontol Clin, 6*:331, 1964.

Moore, Mary Virginia: Binary communication for the severely handicapped. *Arch Phys Med Rehabil, 53(11)*:532, 1972.

Moser, Doris: An understanding approach to the aphasic patient. *Am J Nurs, 61(4)*:52, 1961.

Norton, Carolyn, and Towne, Carol C.: Occupational therapy for aphasic patients. *Am J Occup Ther, 12(6)*:506, 1968.

Olsen, Janice Z., and May, Bella J.: Family education: Necessary adjunct to total stroke rehabilitation. *Am J Occup Ther, 22(2)*:88, 1966.

Overs, Robert P., and Belknap, Elston L.: Educating stroke patient families. *J Chronic Dis, 20(1)*:45, 1967.

Pannbacker, Mary: Publications for families of adult aphasics: A review of the literature. *Rehabil Lit, 33(3)*:72, 1972.

Patrick, Geraldine: Forgotten patients on the medical ward. *Can Nurs, 68(3)*:27, 1972.

Pause, Barbara E., and McCroskey, Robert L.: Treatment of the adult hemiplegic patient with aphasia. *J Am Phys Ther, 42(2)*:111, 1962.

Reeves, Elizabeth W.: The aphasic patient. *Nurs Outlook, 11(7)*:522, 1963.

Rolnick, Michael, and Hopps, H. Ray: Aphasia as seen by the aphasic *J Speech Hear Disord, 34(1)*:48, 1969.

Sands, Elaine, Sarno, Martha Taylor, and Shankweiler, Donald: Long-term assessment of language function in aphasia due to stroke. *Arch Phys Med Rehabil, 50(4)*:202, 1969.

Sarno, John E., and Sarno, Martha Taylor: The diagnosis of speech disorders in brain damaged adults. *Med Clin North Am, 53(3)*:561, 1969.

Sarno, John E., and Sarno, Martha Taylor: *Stroke — the Condition and the Patient*. New York, McGraw, 1969.

Sarno, John E. Swisher, Linda Peck, and Sarno, Martha Taylor: Aphasia in a congenitally deaf man. *Cortex, 5(40*:398, 1969.

Sarno, Martha Taylor: *Aphasia — Selected Readings*. New York, Appleton, 1972.

Sarno, Martha Taylor, and Sands, Elaine: An objective method for the evaluation of speech therapy in aphasia. *Arch Phys Med Rehabil, 51(1)*:49, 1970.

Sarno, Martha Taylor, Silverman, Marla, and LeVita, Eric: Psychosocial factors and recovery in geriatric patients with severe aphasia. *J Am Geriatr Soc, 18(5)*:405, 1970.

Schuell, Hildred, Jenkins, James, and Jimenez-Pabon, Edward: *Aphasia in Adults*. New York, Har-Row, 1964.

Shaw, Bernice L.: Revoluation in stroke care. *RN, 33(1)*:56, 1970.

Smith, Betty Jo, and DeBenneville, Alice K.: An investigation by a visiting nurse association of a home training program for adults with speech and language problems resulting from cerebral vascular accidents and other chronic diseases. *Nurs Res, 16(3)*:310, 1967.

Taylor, Martha L.: *Understanding Aphasia: A Guide for Family and Friends*. New York, Institute of Physical Medicine and Rehabilitation, NYU — Bellevue Medical Center, 1958.

Taylor, Martha L., and Marks, Morton M.: *Aphasia Rehabilitation Manual and Therapy Kit*. New York, McGraw, 1959.

Turner, Gwendolyn E.: The cerebral vascular accident patient. *Nurs Outlook, 8(6)*:326, 1960.

Twamley, R., and Emerick, L.: The nurse's role in aphasia. *Today's Speech, 18(1)*:30, 1970.

Ullman, Montague: *Behavioral Changes in Patients Following Strokes*.

Springfield, Thomas, 1962.

U.S. Dept. of Health, Education and Welfare: *The Vocational Rehabilitation Problems of the Patient with Aphasia.* Washington, D.C., U.S. Dept. of Health, Education and Welfare, Social and Rehabilitation Service, Rehabilitation Services Administration, 1967.

Wepman, Joseph M.: Aphasia — Diagnostic description and thearap. *Hearing and Speech News, 36(1)*3, 1968.

Wepman, Joseph M.: Aphasia therapy: A new look. *J Speech Hear Disord, 37(2)*:203, 1972.

Hemiplegia

Adams, G. F.: Problems in the treatment of hemiplegia. *Gerontol Clin, 9*:285, 1967.

Adams, G. F., and Hurwitz, L. J.: Mental barriers to recovery from strokes. *Lancet, 2*:533, 1963.

Bardach, Joan L.: Psychological factors in hemiplegia. *J Am Phys Ther, 43(11)*:792, 1963.

Bonner, Charles D., *et al.*: The team approach to hemiplegia. *Postgrad Med, 40*:708, 1966.

Boone, Daniel R., and Landes, Bernard A.: Left-right discrimination in hemiplegic patients. *Arch Phys Med Rehabil, 49(96)*:533, 1968.

Butfield, E.: Treatment of acquired speech and language disorders associated with hemiplegia. *Physiotherapy, 52(10)*:350, 1966.

DeBrisay, Amy N., and Stuart, C. Keith: Restoration of communication in the elderly, with special reference to hemiplegic patients: Interim report on program. *J Am Geriatr Soc, 12(7)*:687, 1964.

Fordyce, Wilbert E., and Jones, Robert H.: The efficacy of oral and pantomime instructions for hemiplegic patients. *Arch Phys Med Rehabil, 47(10)*:676, 1966.

Fowler, Roy S. Jr., and Fordyce, Wilbert E.: Adapting care for the brain-damaged patient.*Am J Nurs, 72(10)*:1832, 1972.

Isaacs, Bernard: Disorders of cerebral cortical function associated with strokes. *Physiotherapy, 52(2)*:40, 1966.

Peszczynski, Mieczyslaw: The rehabilitation potential of the late adult hemiplegic. *Am J Nurs, 63(4)*:111, 1963.

Wisconsin State Board of Health: *Bed Activities, Transfers, and Walking for the Hemiplegic Patient.* Madison, Wisconsin State Board of Health, undated pamphlet No. 1000-06.

Wisconsin State Board of Health: *Bed Positioning and Maintenance of Joint Motion for the Hemiplegic Patient.* Madison, Wisconsin State Board of Health, undated pamphlet No. 3000-04.

Wisconsin Division of Health: *Self-care Activities for the Hemiplegic Patient.* Madison, Wisconsin Division of Health, undated pamphlet 3000-08.

Left Hemiplegia

Anderson, Elisabeth K., and Choy, Eugenia: Parietal lobe syndromes in hemiplegia. *Am J Occup Ther, 24(1)*:13, 1970.

Bonkowski, Robert J.: Verbal and extraverbal components of language as related to lateralized brain damage. *J Speech Hear Res, 10(3)*:558, 1967.

Boone, Daniel R.: Communication skills and intelligence in right and left hemiplegics.. *J Speech Hear Disord, 24(3)*:241, 1959.

Hague, Harriet Ruth: An investigation of abstract behavior in patients with cerebral vascular accidents. *Am J Occup Ther, 13(2)*:83, 1959.

Karlin, Isaac W., Eisenson, Jon, Hirschenfang, Samuel, and Miller, Maurice H.: A multi-evaluation study of aphasic and non-aphasic right hemiplegic patients. *J Speech Hear Disord, 24(4)*: 369, 1959.

Knapp, M. E.: Results of language tests of patients with hemiplegia. *Arch Phys Med Rehabil, 43(7)*:317, 1962.

Stovall, Janice D.: Speech therapy implications of CVA's left side. *Nursing Dial Access — Tape No. 506* (Transcript from Wisconsin Division of Health).

Taylor, Mary M.: Analysis of dysfunction in left hemiplegia following stroke. *Am J Occup Ther, 22(6)*:512, 1968.

Chapter 6

PARKINSONISM

ONE of the so-called diseases of middle age or late life with which the speech pathologist may reasonably be expected to work is the problem known as Parkinson's disease. Parkinsonism is estimated to affect "about one percent of the population over 50 years of age" (Mueller, 1971). In 1965, it was estimated that there were over one million victims of this disease in the United States.

Study of the literature available suggests this is not truly a single specific disease but, instead, is a syndrome of signs and symptoms. Because of its varying etiology, the descriptive terms *parkinsonism* or *parkinsonian syndrome* appear to be the most widely acceptable designations. The term *parkinsonism* is used in this book. It refers to patients who exhibit symptoms of tremor, rigidity, and abnormal slowness of movement.

The pattern of additional symptoms is quite different for different patients with the same diagnosis. To date, both the specific etiologies and the pathologies of the disease remain obscure, although the symptoms are believed by many to be associated with widespread lesions in the basal ganglia and/or brain stem. The disorder progresses gradually over a prolonged course until the patient ultimately becomes completely incapacitated.

One of the first symptoms is tremor which usually appears initially in the limbs, particularly the hands. These tremors begin in a rhythmic fashion and are very slight. Over time, there is a gradual increase in intensity of the tremors and a spreading throughout the body. However, the tremors subside on active voluntary movement or complete relaxation. Soon muscular rigidity develops along with a slowness and poverty of movements. The patient assumes a particular stooped position. Eventually impairment of various movements causes a rapid, shuffling, *tiptoe* gait which passes from a walking to a running pace. The face assumes a masklike appearance.

Each Parkinson patient is different. They do not all have identical problems but could have one or more of the following with respect to the oral and phonatory areas: Some will dribble saliva (particularly those whose round-shouldered stoop is accompanied by additional drooping of the head). Some do not chew, thereby presenting nutritional problems. There may be difficulty with the epiglottis, hence an ever-present problem of both foods and liquids getting caught in the larynx. Despite an intense fear of choking, the patient must be urged to eat and drink. Defecation problems may also accompany the eating impairments.

Many of these patients develop a forward pitch and a shuffling gait. Because they fall frequently, precautions must be taken. However, it is believed that the patients should not be strapped in a wheelchair, but rather be allowed to walk around freely. A major goal is to keep them moving.

With respect to speech, the features of rigidity, tremor, and abnormal slowness of movement can affect all aspects of the speaking function. The rounded shoulders, effecting partial collapse of the rib cage, interferes with optimal respiration; the patient may be unable to generate sufficient amounts of aerodynamic energy for normal phonation and articulation. As a result, the voice weakens and fades to a whisper. There is an inability to sustain phonation. In addition, the speech pattern becomes too regular and monotonous: pitch inflections and normal stress patterns are lost; rhythm is seriously disturbed. Often the rate of speaking is increased. "Some patients manifest a propulsive, festinating type of speech with deteriorating intelligibility as speech progresses" (Darley, 1963).

Articulation movements can become so delimited as to result in a dysarthric, unintelligible mumbling. The patient may be able to repeat words and phrases clearly during therapy, but be unable to transfer this clarity to spontaneous communication outside the therapy room. Such disparity between clinical performance and functional performance has led at least one speech pathologist to advocate functional evaluation (see Sarno, 1968).

Whatever intervention techniques are attempted, it must be recognized that they are merely palliative — not corrective — and can only hope to delay the progression of the syndrome. To maintain the status quo is a real achievement. Care plans can include a large armamentarium of drugs, and must include tremendous amounts of psychological support. The patient and his relatives must be fully educated in the failing aspects of parkinsonism. They must understand that mental illness is not involved. Intellectual faculties usually remain unimpaired. The patient remains alert, and understands, even to the ultimate progression of total *freezing*. They must know that parkinsonism is a continually progressive deterioration and that motivation remains the key to the success of any type of care plan.

While the preceding ideas reflect the major thrust of the present-day literature's views of parkinsonism, one should not overlook recent experimental findings (Reitan and Boll) which found twenty-five individuals with parkinsonism (when compared with a control group matched for sex, race, age, and education) to be "significantly impaired across a broad range of additional adaptive abilities which are not dependent on the adequacy of motor performance" (Reitan and Boll, 1971). Accordingly, Reitan and Boll cautioned that lack of or reduction of cognitive ability may be the critical missing factor rather than lack of motivation. Should these researchers' findings prove to be representative of great numbers of individuals with parkinsonism, the implications for rehabilitation programs are profound and the widely-held assumption of *unimpaired intellectual facility* would need to be seriously reconsidered.

Within the past decade or so, operations have been considerably successful on the rigidity and tremor. Such surgery is usually directed at creating a lesion in the thalamus. However, not all persons afflicted with parkinsonism are suitable surgery candidates. Extenuating factors include age, mental and physical status, rate of progression of the disease, degree of bradykinesia (abnormal slowness of movement), and the presence of other disease. Unfortunately, surgery appears to have little beneficial effect on speech.

Another major treatment involved in parkinsonism is that of chemotherapy. Those interested in a detailed listing of the various drugs that have been used can find presentations of drug types, daily dosages, symptoms affected, and side effects in the book *Parkinson's Disease* by Barbeau, Doshay, and Spiegel.

The most recent drug which has had rather spectacular effects in some cases (and no effect in others) is Levodopa, commonly referred to as L-dopa. It seems presumptuous of the present author to try to summarize the pros and cons on the use of L-dopa. The greatest gains appear to be in relieving the rigidity and improving the patient's gait and masklike appearance. Because L-dopa can give rise to extremely serious side effects, the drug is usually administered only to hospitalized cases. Side effects include anorexia (lack or loss of the appetite for food), nausea, weakness, sweating, hypersexuality, changes in blood pressure, dizziness, cardiac arhythmia, restlessness, hallucinations, delusions, aggressive outbursts, insomnia, and mood swings (from elevation to depression and back).

Maintenance therapies for parkinsonism must be orientated and implemented around activities of daily living. Such therapeutic efforts include postural retraining and are directed to the prevention of stiffening and contracture of joints. Physical therapy approaches are based on maintaining independence of movement that will allow continuing social contacts.

Apparently surgical therapy does not in any way obviate continuing the use of all other forms of treatment. Monotony of voice, difficulty in swallowing, and excessive salivation are not normally benefited by surgery. The need remains for chewing and swallowing and respiratory maintenance therapy.

It is possible that chewing and swallowing techniques may not be considered as routine speech pathology activities by some of the readers of this book. Originally, the author shared such doubts until he became aware of the various ways that different health professionals viewed these activities. If chewing and swallowing is not worked with by the nurse, the occupational therapist, or the physical therapist, then this need will undoubtedly remain unmet unless the speech pathologist assumes this responsibility. This he can certainly do, recognizing the substrata required for verbal communication. The same musculature used in speaking functions for chewing and swallowing as well. Ideally, chewing and swallowing techniques are pursued in cooperation with members of the nursing staff.* Where team efforts at maintenance therapy are nonexistent or cannot be developed, the speech pathologist must depend on his own knowledge in helping to maintain speech at the present level of efficiency.

The slogan "Keep them moving" applies to eating, as well as to the grosser movements involved in posture, locomotion, etc. Jaws, lips, and tongue are exercised in excessive teeth-grinding movements while eating. If such efforts prove too distasteful socially, the patient might prefer to eat in his own room rather than in the dining room. Chewing gum several times a day — geriodontists would insist on the sugarless varieties — is also helpful. Further tongue exercise is afforded by the action of cleaning between the gum ridges and cheeks, not only after each meal, but between meals as well. Besides the tongue activities involved in such cleaning, the tongue can also participate in opposition exercises with the lips — i.e. pushing the tongue forward, while restraining it, with the lips, from popping out.

Similarly, the tongue can be pushed out against the cheek. Additional hand resistance against the cheek can be supplied by either the patient himself, or a staff member, pushing the tongue back within the dental arches.

Some of the tongue techniques long in use with young cerebral palsied children are also applicable with parkinsonism. These include the *removal behaviors* the tongue automatically assumes upon the placement of foreign matter in the mouth. The noncrunchy type of peanut butter, and thick, sticky jams are useful when positioned on the alveolar ridge, or when placed between teeth and cheek, or between teeth and lips. Such activities can also be mediated with successively coarser foodstuffs such as small pieces of dry cereals, crackers, and toast. The size and consistency of the foods are as important as the method of utilization. In any of the techniques utilizing foods, it is wise to

*Specific techniques for improving drinking and swallowing and chewing and swallowing abilities of adults with oral paralysis are available as numbers 1 and 2 in a series published by the Section of Patient Care Practices, Wisconsin Division of Health. The same source further augments such assistance with Tape 507 on *Oral Paralysis,* a printed transcription of which is also available.

ascertain in advance whether or not the patient refused that type of food in the past. Also, one should always be apprised of whether or not a diabetic condition is present — precluding the use of such foods as nondiabetic gum drops unless cleared by the attending physician.

Blowing, sucking, and yawning can also be utilized in an exercise regimen. Alternately grinning and puckering can exercise the lips. A way of checking up on the patient and his chewing efforts is to leave a gumdrop in his mouth for a few minutes. If it remains whole when retrieved, there is strong reason to suspect his chewing efforts are diminishing.

Attempts to work against the clenched jaw and closed mouth include sustaining vowel sounds, particularly those requiring the greatest jaw opening such as *ah* and the vowel sound in *and*. Various devices might be utilized to chart the changing durations of the patient's open-mouthed phonation time. Patients should also be encouraged to overexaggerate, for several short periods every day, all oral movements while talking.

Once a nursing staff realizes that these oral activities can help to stave off the progressive deterioration of parkinsonism, and that such delay will not only help the patient, but will lighten their nursing roles in feeding and drinking activities, they are apt to participate wholeheartedly in these activities, freeing the speech pathologist to tackle other problems.

With respect to the respiratory problems accompanying parkinsonism, any speech pathologist well-trained in the basics of voice and speech production should know how to proceed. It is easy to understand how the shoulder rounding delimits vital capacity of the lungs. Excessive interference with the rising-falling activity of the rib cage will ultimately result in a weakening of the voice.

The combination of reduced vital capacity and unresolved dietary problems can lead to constipation — so characteristic of individuals with parkinsonism. Hopefully, interaction of the speech pathologist with the nutritionist and the physician can minimize the reliance on soft, liquid diets which only serve to aggravate the chewing problems. The possibility of utilizing coarser foods, such as melba toast and raw vegetables, increases the possibility of exercising the eating/speaking musculature.

Insight into the drinking habits of the patient is also required. Is he attempting to flush down his food, rather than chewing it well? Once we all understand our mutual interdependency in total patient care, the nurse, nutritionist, physical therapist, occupational therapist, and speech pathologist can work to further each other's goals while pursuing activities unique to their own profession.

The adverse effect upon respiration of shoulder-rounding would seem to call into question the wisdom of using the type of wheelchair which has a rounded or collapsible back. Instead, it is best for patients with parkinsonism to sit in straight-back chairs. In advanced cases requiring bracing and typing, it would be well for a wide piece of material to be used to hold the shoulders back. Once the patient understands the reason for these procedures, he is ready to cooperate. What a pity that so many of our cases have things done to them without explanation of the benefits to be derived! Other things being equal, these patients understand, and will assist all of us if they realize the delaying, maintaining purposes of our techniques. Explanation, when accompanied by demonstration, should bring about maximum cooperation. It is amazing how many of these patients, given such treatment, change from being *difficult, cranky, crotchety old men* to patients that everyone is happy to assist.

An exercise designed to delay respiratory deterioration is to have the patient sit with bent elbows at his side, while holding his hands up near his shoulders, palms facing forward. The staff member momentarily pushes against the patient's hands while the patient resists the movement, simultaneously producing sound (such as "ah"). A modification which the patient can do by himself is to lean forward with rigid arms, placing his weight on his hands on a stable tabletop. He phonates (makes a vowel sound) while putting his weight on his hands. Efforts to maintain adequate loudness include increasing the distance between the speech pathologist and the patient. For example the pathologist, outside the room, says "Tell me to come into the room so I can hear you."

Another aid to better respiration is the use of blow bottles. This is recommended not only for Parkinson patients, but for individuals with multiple sclerosis as well. Although blow bottles are commercially available through medical supply houses, it is certainly a simple thing to create some of your own if you are a do-it-yourself type of person. Two bottles and some tubing are the major ingredients.

In the author's home community one young multiple sclerotic housewife keeps a set of blow bottles in her kitchen. As she says: "Whenever I pass the bottles, I take a blow." This very intelligent young woman, who has a master's degree in speech pathology, was unable to refer to any research literature supporting the beneficial effects of blow bottle use for multiple sclerosis or parkinsonism, but she said "I cannot believe that with my multiple sclerosis, I could be swimming a half mile daily, as I do at the present time, were it not for my extended period of use of the blow bottles in my attempt to maintain sufficient respiratory skill to adequately serve speech."

It is cases such as these that suggest the desperate need for speech pathologists, nurses, and occupational and physical therapists to share rehabilitation methods and techniques. Such sharing is definitely not achieved without the possibility of some problems. These problems are most apt to arise if any of the cooperating professionals is insecure in his own work.

Parkinsonism is rarely listed as a cause of death. However, parkinsonian individuals are more susceptible to the killing illnesses, such as pneumonia. As the Parkinson deterioration progresses upwards in the body, the speech pathologist may need to work out systems of alternate communication for the total staff to utilize when verbalization becomes impossible. With the so-called completely *frozen* Parkinson case, *yes-no* responses are mediated by eye blinks. Pointers (including flashlight beams) can be attached to head bands of patients still possessing head movements for use with communication boards consisting of pictures, words, alphabet letters, and/or numbers.

In summary, speech management of the Parkinson case includes attention to phonatory problems related to respiration (particularly to fading loudness level), to problems of speaking rate, and to labored articulation. All such problems have a direct relationship to reasonably functioning musculature — the same muscles with which the physical and occupational therapists are likely to be working.

REFERENCES

Barbeau, Andre, Doshay, Lewis, and Spiegel, Ernest A.: *Parkinson's Disease: Trends in Research and Treatment.* New York, Grune, 1965.

Darley, Frederic L.: Speech problems in the aging. *Postgrad Med, 33(3)*:298, 1963.

Mueller, Peter B.: Parkinson's disease: Motor-speech behavior in a selected group of patients. *Folia Phoniatr, 23(5)*:333, 1971.

Reitan, Ralph M., and Boll, Thomas J.: Intellectual and cognitive functions in Parkinson's disease. *J Consult Clin Psychol, 37(3)*:364, 1971.

Sarno, Martha Taylor: Speech impairment in Parkinson's disease. *Arch Phys Med Rehabil, 49(5)*:269, 1968.

ADDITIONAL READING LIST

American Medical Association: The cripplers — Parkinson's disease. *Today's Health, 43(8)*:34, 1965.

Buck, Joyce Felstein, and Cooper, Irving S.: Speech problems in parkinsonian patients undergoing anterior choroidal artery occlusion or chemopallidectomy. *Am Geriatr Soc, 4(12)*:1285, 1956.

Canter, Gerald J.: Speech characteristics of patients with Parkinson's disease: I. Intensity, pitch, and duration. *J Speech Hear Disord, 28(3)*:221, 1963.

Canter, Gerald J.: Speech characteristics of patients with Parkinson's disease. II. Physiological support for speech. *J Speech Hear Disord, 30(1)*:44, 1965.

Canter, Gerald J.: Speech characteristics of patients with Parkinson's disease: III. Articulation, diadochokinesis, and over-all speech adequacy. *J Speech Hear Disord, 3)(30)*:217, 1965.

Carroll, Bettie: Fingers to toes. *Am J Nurs, 71(3)*:550, 1971.

Cotzias, George C., Papavasiliou, Paul S., and Gellene, Rosemary: Modification of parkinsonism — chronic treatment with L-Dopa. *N Engl J Med, 280(7)*:337, 1969.

Fangman, Anne, and O'Malley, William E.: L-Dopa and the patient with Parkinson's disease. *Am J Nurs, 69(7)*:1455, 1969.

Greene, M. C. L., and Watson, B. W.: The value of speech amplification in Parkinson's disease patients. *Folia Phoniatr, 20(4)*:250, 1968.

Jerger, J., Mier, M., Boshes, B., and Canter, G.: Auditory behavior in Parkinsonism. *Acta Otolaryngol, 52*:541, 1960.

Mawdsley, C., and Gamsu, C. V.: Periodicity of speech in Parkinsonism. *Nature (Lond), 231(5301)*:315, 1971.

Merritt, H. H.: Paralysis agitans (Parkinson's syndrome). In Merritt, H.

Houston (Ed.): *A Textbook of Neurology,* 4th ed. Philadelphia, Lea & Febiger, 1967.

Morrison, Eleanor B., Rigrodsky, Seymour, and Mysak, Edward D.: Parkinson's disease: Speech disorder and released infantile oroneuromotor activity. *J Speech Hear Res, 13(3)*:655, 1970.

Rigrodsky, Seymour, and Morrison, Eleanor B.: Speech changes in Parkinsonism during L-Dopa therapy: Preliminary findings. *J Am Geriatr Soc, 18(2)*:142, 1970.

Tyler, Eunice: Management of Parkinson's disease with L-Dopa therapy. *Can Nurs, 67(4)*:41, 1971.

Wisconsin Division of Health, Section of Patient Care Practices: *Number 1 in a series — Exercises to Improve the Drinking and Swallowing Ability of an Adult With Oral Paralysis.*Madison, Wisconsin Division of Health.

Wisconsin Division of Health, Section of Patient Care Practices: *Number 2 in a series — Exercises to Improve the Chewing and Swallowing Ability of an Adult with Oral Paralysis.* Madison, Wisconsin Division of Health.

Chapter 7

MULTIPLE SCLEROSIS

MULTIPLE sclerosis (commonly referred to as MS) is "a disease of obscure etiology, characterized clinically by symptoms indicating the presence of multiple lesions in the white matter of the brain and spinal cord" (Harrison, *et al.,* 1966). It remains today, a century and a third after it was first described, a "demyelinating disease with an unknown cause, an unexplained geographic distribution, an unpredictable course, an undiscovered cure and without a simple laboratory test to confirm its diagnosis" (National Multiple Sclerosis Society, 1969b) Accordingly, Miller notes that "diagnosis can hardly ever be regarded as absolutely certain short of necropsy findings" (Miller, 1964). No single infallible sign or symptom can be pinpointed. It has an unpredictable course, varying widely in its modes of progression. It has ups and downs and periods of stability.

Its beginning symptoms, such as visual blurring, double vision, or tingling in one of the limbs, can be nothing more than a slight inconvenience. Symptoms typically come and go. Remissions may last several months, several years. It proceeds from remissions to acute exacerbations (increase in the severity of any symptoms or disease) to further remissions with increasing residual effects each time. Sometimes symptoms persist with no improvement. It varies widely from individual to individual in the number of symptoms, their order of occurrence, the body area affected, and the intensity of their occurrence. It is difficult to foretell the course of the disease — some multiple sclerotics are almost completely incapacitated, while some resume near-normal activities. Average life expectancy after onset is more than twenty-five years.

"Signs and symptoms (of MS) may be transient" (Poser, *et al.,* 1966), causing difficulty in clinical diagnosis. The signs and symptoms include ocular disturbances (diplopia, blurred vision, diminution of visual acuity, visual field defects, etc.). muscle weakness, gait ataxia, nonequilibratory disturbances (intention tremor, dysdiadochokinesia, incoordination of fine movements, etc.), dysarthria (neither cortical in origin nor due to local conditions such as vocal cord paralysis), urinary disturbances, parasthesias (any spontaneous subjective disturbance of sensation). "The real problem seems to lie with the fact that symptoms, as well as neurologic signs, may be evanescent and mild enough so that medical advice may not be sought by the patient unless some moderately severe degree of functional disability occurs" (Poser, *et al.*, 1966).

The age of onset normally is between twenty and forty years of age, with first symptoms appearing in one out of five cases before the age of twenty. It rarely develops before eighteen or after forty-five years of age. Its incidence is five to six times greater in cold, damp, northern climates than in the South. However, the disease cannot be cured by moving from a cold to a warmer climate. It appears slightly more frequently in females than males. It occurs more frequently in Europe than in the United States, but it is rare in Africa and Asia.

The etiology has not yet been validated, but there are three causal hypotheses which appear to be the most promising. According to these, it is either (1) due to a slow-acting respiratory virus infection, (2) the result of an autoimmune response to an exogenous factor (i.e., an allergy), or (3) an autoimmune response to an endogenous substance, possibly produced in the brain or spinal cord, that keeps the disease process going. These possibilities are clarified and elaborated upon by Bardossi (1971).

The disease produces a structural change in the nervous system. Patches of scar tissue develop throughout the brain and spinal cord. Normally, nerve fibers are encased in a fatty-like substance called myelin. It is believed that this substance acts like insulation on an electric wire, to protect the nerves that transmit electrical impulses. In the MS process, there is a scattered disintegration of bits of myelin. The lost insulation is replaced by scar (sclerotic) tissue. Remissions are thought to be due to regeneration of the sclerotic myelin. While only the myelin sheath is affected, nerve impulses can be transmitted, but with reduced effectiveness. Once the nerve fiber itself has been replaced by scar tissue in progressive stages of the disease, transmission of impulses stops, and there can be no recovery of the functions affected.

Exacerbation and progression of the disease appear to be set off or accentuated by "general poor health, generalized infection, illness with fever, too much exertion or undue fatigue, injuries, allergic diseases, and emotional upsets" (AMA, 1965).

Since MS affects people in the prime of life, evaluations by physical and occupational therapy are mandatory in order to determine the patient's total capacity to engage in work, as well as activities of daily living.

The standard physical therapy evaluation is augmented by "a separate specific physical capacities appraisal. This consists of a series of critical physical factors in job performance. Such factors as pushing, pulling, lifting, carrying, etc. are considered" (Aldes, 1967).

The occupational therapy evaluation "comprises prevocational testing, activities of daily living, and job sample activity (work simulation) which are valuable in the total occupational assessment. Included is aptitude testing where specific occupational validity has been established, rather than generalized testing with only remote occupational relationship. Each of these disciplines is needed to complete the total assessment of potential occupational goals" (Aldes, 1967).

An exceptionally valuable publication for basic, practical suggestions for everyday activities is that prepared by Laura M. Braunel, Carole A. James, and Janice D. Stovall entitled *MS is a Family Affair.* This publication of the National Easter Seal Society for Crippled Children and Adults abounds in *how-to-do-it* aids, all of which are printed in large-size type, and clear, simple language. Additional adaptations of the home to accommodate the patient's problems appear in the 1968 article by Plummer, and in *Homemaking for the Handicapped* (May, Wagonor, and Batzke, 1966). Further pertinent information can be found in *Mealtime Manual for the Aged and Handicapped* (Klinger, Frieden, and Sullivan, 1970).

The best treatment procedures at present appear to consist of building up general resistance, avoiding fatigue and exposure to extremes of hot and cold, eliminating exposure to infection with vigorous treatment when infection does occur, avoiding other factors that may bring on relapses, obtaining sufficient rest and nutritious meals, and remaining under a physician's care to prevent infection and control distressing symptoms. Needless to say, each treatment program must be "highly individualized depending on the patient's medical status, needs, and problems" (Marks, 1959).

While these procedures are obviously intended to counteract complications as well as to directly treat the presumed basic disease process, the patient is undoubtedly most assisted by the treatment of symptoms. "Such therapy is directed toward the amelioration of motor dysfunction, the alleviation of bladder and rectal dysfunction, minor help for visual disturbances, reduction of pain, and improvement of pernicious emotional reactions and mood disorders" (Schumacher, 1970).

As the disease progresses, the patient is limited by lack of endurance. Spontaneity of living must be sacrificed in favor of scheduling every activity of the day, including the all-important rest periods. Swimming in quiet, warm water is an excellent means of exercise. Use of a golf cart for transportation (to grocery store, church, library, school, etc.) can help to maintain a degree of independence.

Many, perhaps most, multiple sclerosis patients appear hopeful and cheerful. They tend to be very nice, seldom arguing or talking back. They have learned that when hostilities are generated, their symptoms will become even worse. Hence they retreat into a cocoon of euphoric cheerfulness which Morton Marks identifies as "probably a psychological defense reaction in a younger individual faced with the prospect of an overwhelming chronic and progressively disabling disorder" (Marks, 1959). Others are "irritable, dissatisfied, tense, apprehensive or depressed" (Schumacher, 1970).

Morton Marks notes, in describing the components of individual rehabilitation programs, that "A careful psychological and social evaluation is imperative. His mental and intellectual status, his personality structure, and his motivation must also be ascertained. Often intensive corrective efforts must be directed to the social and psychological factors rather than to the physical disability itself if significant benefit is to be anticipated from the rehabilitation program" (Marks, 1959).

Of equal if not of greater importance is the complex family relationship roles and responsibilities. Total family resources "should be pooled and devoted to insistence on a full and useful life for each member" (National Multiple Sclerosis Society, 1969a). "The patient is plagued with questions about changed appearance, dependency, adequacy as a spouse or parent" (National Multiple Sclerosis Society, 1969a). It is well for relatives, neighbors, and friends to bear in mind that a crippled body in no way implies crippled intelligence. Likewise one would not presume a termination of sexual relations. The patient is not devoid of sexual desires and drives, but modifications are required. MS does not equate with cessation of sex!

Since a definite prognosis is impossible, the patient must reduce or nullify his fear of death and focus on day-to-day life. The more that all members of the family understand the condition, the less chance there is of family disagreements. In some cases, the patient's abominable behavior — even though he attempts to control it — stretches all normal concepts of understanding.

Patient and family instability can be negated or minimized by a set of realistic goals. The patient must experience a reduced pressure to perform all activities. Yet, he must feel he is needed. For the married female patient, sit-down work such as bill paying, checkbook balancing, menu planning, can replace the greater demands of the housewife's cleaning activities. It does not help for the patient's mate to say "Rest and have a good day" while expecting a clean house, clean clothes, and gourmet meals.

Because speech changes seldom occur until MS is well advanced, the speech pathologist rarely participates in rehabilitation programs directed toward returning the patient to employment. However, to the extent that speech problems develop in advanced stages of MS, speech can be said to become slow, slurred, monotonous, with irregular pauses and significant loudness decreases. This combination of speech disruptions gave rise to Grewel's 1957 term "dysarthro-pneumo-phonia" (Ewanowski, 1970).

Perhaps, then, it is most meaningful to discuss the relationship of speech to increasing dysfunction of such processes as respiration, phonation, articulation, and audition. Because the lesions of MS are primarily of the white matter of the brain and spinal cord, and less frequently encroach upon the grey matter, there seldom are psychological, intellectual, and symbolic language deficits. Since there is seldom gross intellectual deterioration or extensive personality change, motivation tends to remain at a high level — sometimes to the extent of the harboring of unrealistic goals.

Respiratory dysfunction may be marked by reduced lung volume and poor control of exhalation, resulting in diminished loudness, and in inadequate supply of outgoing air to sustain longer phrases and sentences. There might also be attempts at speaking on inhalation — frequently related to problems of inhaling food.

Phonatory dysfunctioning may lead to *odd* sounding vocal quality (due to aperiodic vibrational patterns), nasal voice quality (due to disturbed resonance characteristics), reduced pitch variability (monotone or severely restricted pitch range), weak voice (already mentioned as related to respiration), and trouble initiating vocal fold vibration (glottal spasticity).

Articulatory functioning may be affected by reduced strength, range of motion, and speed of articulator movement, resulting in slow, sluggish, imprecise sound production. A scanning of lalling type of speech can occur due to prolonged phonation accompanied by slurred articulation of the consonant sound, accompanied by abnormal pitch level and inflection. The dysarthric speech can arise from poor coordination among the articulators and between articulatory, phonatory, and respiratory systems.

Research on the hearing of MS patients presents a confusing picture. The literature reports both conductive and sensorineural types of loss, as well as no hearing losses related specifically to the disease. Possibly the best justified conclusion for the time being is that advanced by LeZak and Selhub to the effect that "there is reason to conclude this population as a whole demonstrates hearing similar to that found in the general population of the same age" (LeZak and Selhub, 1966).

Speech intelligibility is adversely affected as progress of MS affects neural impairment to the muscles used for talking and eating, producing weakness and incoordination. A functional overlay of disuse atrophy, if present, will also contribute to greater speech dysfunction. Any improvement lies in the functional utilization of the patient's remaining capacities, rather than in remission of symptoms or any lessening of the organic impairment.

Farmakides and Boone noted that "the most effective technique in improving speech for these persons was the age-old advice of asking the patient to speak louder, often producing immediately more normal rhythm, less nasality and sharper articulation. (Farmakides and Boone, 1960). However, the authors also advocate speech activities involving control of exhalation and direct work upon sound production stressing control and direction. Certainly phrasing (and related breathing) techniques would also assist in gaining greater vocal control.

In a paper presented in 1970 at an MS conference in Madison, Wisconsin, Dr. Stanley J. Ewanowski advanced five criteria for selecting patients with MS for speech therapy. They are "(1) absence of cerebral involvement; (2) no, or limited, personality changes; (3) no gross intellectual deterioration; (4) presence of long remissive periods; and (5) motivation at a high level" (Ewanowski, 1970). He concluded that the more of these factors present in any given patient, the better the prognosis for improving speech communication.

In the final analysis, the speech pathologist recognizes the following as indicative of the need for speech pathology services: spasticity, *open mouth,* weak voice, nystagmus, speaking on inhalation, short attention span, and unrealistic goals. He wants something done to challenge chewing at each meal. Related therapy includes talking with teeth closed but with lips open, and talking while pretending to chew with the lips open. The speech pathologist is also interested in improving vital capacity (breathing). Some patients find the use of blow bottles helpful.

For the most severely involved cases having only neck movement left, a headband flashlight can be used to point to need words or pictures, or to letters of the alphabet in spelling his needs.

Any discussion of MS would be grossly incomplete without reference to the pioneering efforts of the National Multiple Sclerosis Society in stimulating, coordinating, and disseminating research findings. The local chapters of this organization work with government agencies and industry to provide gainful employment. They make available *talking books* for patients unable to read or to hold and turn pages of a book. They provide transportation, equipment and aids, counseling, homemaker service, and referrals for medical and nursing care. They provide companionship and social events (picnics, parties, theatre, and sporting events). They provide friendly visiting and home care arrangements, plus professional counseling. (See *MS*, No. VI BR 45 2/69 100M of the National MS Society, 257 Park Avenue South, New York, N.Y. 10010). In addition, they maintain sizeable listings of publications and motion pictures available for the edification of professionals and other concerned individuals.

REFERENCES

Aldes, John H.: Rehabilitation of multiple sclerosis patients. *J Rehabil, 33(2)*:10, 1967.

American Medical Association: The cripplers: Multiple sclerosis. *Today's Health, 43(8)*:36, 1965.

Bardossi, Fulvio: *Multiple Sclerosis: Grounds for Hope*. New York, Public Aff Comm (Public Affairs Pamphlet No. 335A), 1971.

Braunel, Laura M., James, Carole A., and Stovall, Janice D.: *MS is a Family Affair*. Chicago, National Easter Seal Society for Crippled Children and Adults, 1972.

Ewanowski, Stanley J.: Speech and language patterns in multiple sclerosis. Paper read at the conference "Multiple Sclerosis 1970: The disease, the patient, the therapeutic environment." Madison, Wisconsin, April 10, 1970.

Farmakides, Mary N., and Boone, Daniel R.: Speech problems of patients with multiple sclerosis. *J Speech Hear Dis, 25(4)*:385, 1960.

Harrison, Tinsley Randolph, *et al.* (Eds.): *Principles of Internal Medicine*, 5th ed. New York, McGraw, 1966.

Klinger, Judith Lannefeld, Frieden, Fred H., and Sullivan, Richard A.: *Mealtime Manual for the Aged and Handicapped*. New York, Essandess,

1970.

Lezak, Raymond J., and Selhub, Shirley: On hearing in multiple sclerosis. *Ann Otol Rhino Laryngol, 75(4)*:1102, 1966.

Marks, Morton: Multiple sclerosis. *Health News of New York State Department of Health,* May, 1959 (revised and reprinted). New York, National Multiple Sclerosis Society, 1970.

May, Elizabeth, Wagonor, Lietha, and Batzke, Elinor: *Homemaking for the Handicapped.* New York, Dodd, 1966.

Miller, Henry: Trauma and multiple sclerosis. *Lancet, 1964(1)*:848, April 18, 1964.

National Multiple Sclerosis Society: *The Clergy and Multiple Sclerosis.* New York, National Multiple Sclerosis Society, 1969a.

National Multiple Sclerosis Society: *Multiple Sclerosis.* New York, National Multiple Sclerosis Society, 1969b.

Plummer, Elizabeth M.: The MS patient. *Am J Nurs, 86(10)*:2161, 1968. (Reprinted and made available by the National Multiple Sclerosis Society.)

Poser, Charles M., Presthus, Jan, and Horsdal, Odd: Clinical characteristics of autopsy-proved multiple sclerosis. *Neurology, 16(8)*:791, 1966.

Schumacher, George A.: Multiple sclerosis. In Conn, Howard F. (Ed.): *Current Therapy, 1970.* Philadelphia, Saunders, 1970.

ADDITIONAL READING LIST

Brookshire, Robert H.: Control of "involuntary" crying behavior emitted by multiple sclerosis patient. *J Commun Disord, 3(3)*:171, 1970.

Brown, Joe R.: Recent studies in multiple sclerosis: Inferences on rehabilitation and employability. *Mayo Clin Proc, 44(10)*:758, 1969.

Darley, Frederic L., Aronson, Arnold E., and Brown, Joe R.: Clusters of deviant speech dimensions in the dysarthrias. *J Speech Hear Res, 12(3)*:462, 1969.

Darley, Frederic L., Brown, Joe R., and Goldstein, Norman P.: Dysarthria in multiple sclerosis. *J Speech Hear Res, 15(2)*:229, 1972.

Dean Geoffrey: The multiple sclerosis problem. *Sci Am, 223(1)*:40, 1970.

DeJong, Russell N.: MS — Crippler of young adults. *Today's Health, 42(11)*: 36, 1964.

Matthews, Jack, Everson, Richard, and Burgi, Ernest J.: Effect of Isoniazid on the speech of multiple sclerosis patients. *J Speech Hear Disord, 25(1)*38, 1960.

Merritt, Hiram Houston: *A Textbook of Neurology,* 5th ed. Philadelphia, Lea & Febiger, 1973.

Simmons, James Q. Jr.: *Multiple Sclerosis and the Practical Nurse.* New York, National Multiple Sclerosis Society, 1972.

Chapter 8

POSTLARYNGECTOMY

FOR the past hundred years, a small but increasing percentage of our population has had to learn to adjust to life without a larynx. The first laryngectomy (total removal of larynx) was performed in 1873 by Bilbroth (Levin, 1940). A long lag in the number of operations followed this pioneering treatment for laryngeal cancer because it was believed the operation shortened life expectancy. This belief is no longer held.

Breathing and speech are dissociated as a result of such surgical removal. Postoperatively the patient breathes through a stoma (opening) into the trachea (windpipe). The previous outflow of air from the lungs no longer exits through the mouth and nose. The most obvious consequence of this operation is the absence of speech.

As serious as this is — the abrupt loss of the patient's primary means for social relationship — there are other sequelae which compound the laryngectomee's problems.

He will probably experience difficulties in swallowing. He will be unable to cough, sneeze, and blow his nose as he used to. He will be unable to whistle, hum, and sing. There will be interference with his sense of smell and of taste. He will be unable to lift heavy objects or strain hard because he cannot lock his breath in, as he formerly could. Defecation may be interfered with. *Normal* childbirth for a laryngectomized woman is no longer possible. Showering becomes a dangerous procedure. Bedclothes may need to be replaced so that wads of lint are not inhaled directly into the lungs. Dusty occupations must be given up.

The consequences of these changes and functions tend to create psychological problems including an *other-worldly* feeling. His self-image is disturbed. He must adjust to new techniques for breathing, lifting, etc. The patient is apt to sink into depression. He may find it difficult to combat the fear of further cancer. The combination of physical, psychological, social, communication, and vocational aspects precludes the possibility that any one professional can help with all of the patient's problems.

Obviously prognosis will depend, to a great extent, on the personality of the laryngectomee. However, certain steps can be taken with all laryngectomees to increase the probability of optimal recovery. Of greatest importance are the matters of preoperative preparation of the patient involving explanation and counseling and predischarge conferencing to prepare the patient to live comfortably as a laryngectomee.

The more the patient understands what is involved, what processes are disrupted, and what compensatory measures can be taken, the greater the possibility of acceptable postoperative adjustment and success. Much counseling is aimed at keeping the patient's attention outside himself — on hobbies, family, vocation, etc.

Predischarge conferencing normally involves the physician, nurse, speech pathologist, social worker, patient, and the patient's family. This consultation deals with such matters as management of the tracheotomy tube and the tracheal fistula; dangers of loose hair, powder and setting sprays in barbershop or beauty shop; design of shirts and dresses; the use of stoma shields; regularity of esophageal speech practice; relationship of excitement, embarrassment, or other disturbing emotions to esophageal speech success; facing the reactions of family, friends, and the general public; and vocational rehabilitation.

It remains a fact that the best attack on total adjustment is through speech reeducation. Two main approaches are available. One is the substitution of esophageal voice; the other is the use of an artificial larynx. Grossly oversimplified, one can describe esophageal speech as that process of shaping, with the oral structures, sequences of controlled burp- or belch-like sounds which the patient learns to make in rapid sequence and to increase in duration. The air is inducted into the upper part of the esophagus; its controlled eructation through the esophagus facilitates a vibration — a substitute for vocal fold vibration.

Goals of the speech pathologist include the avoidance of (1) unnecessary lip movements, (2) loud blowing sounds from the tracheal opening, (3) noisy swallowing attempts, (4) reversion to whispered speech, and (5) patient satisfaction with poor articulation.

Speech pathologists tend to discourage the use of an electrolarynx until it is established beyond any reasonable doubt that the patient is unable to achieve speech through the use of his remaining throat and esophageal structures. The electrolarynx has the disadvantages of being conspicuous, noisy, unnatural sounding, and subject to mechanical failure or breakdown. It requires the use of a hand and calls attention to the user's disability.

In addition to the crucial personnel of physician, speech pathologist, nurse, and social worker, most rehabilitative efforts draw heavily upon the assistance of other laryngectomees who are successful esophageal speakers and upon structured group interaction therapy programs to facilitate life adjustment as a laryngectomee. Where available the patient becomes a member of the local *Lost Chord, Anamilo,* or *New Voice* clubs. The sole purpose of these clubs is to help laryngectomees. The clubs are affiliated with the International Association of Laryngectomees under sponsorship of the American Cancer Society.

REFERENCES

Levin, Nathaniel M.: Teaching the laryngectomized patient to talk. *Arch Otolaryngol, 32*:299, 1940.

ADDITIONAL READING LIST

Adler, Sol: Speech after laryngectomy. *Am J Nurs, 69(9)*:2138, 1969.

Anonymous: An electronic larynx lets patient convert "buzz" into speech. *JAMA, 206(8)*:1710, 1968.

Bangs, Jack L., Lierle, D. M., and Strother, C. R.: Speech after laryngectomy. *J Speech Disord, 11(3)*:171, 1946.

Damste, Helbert: Rehabilitation after laryngectomy. *Rehabil Lit, 27(9)*:266, 1966.

De St. Andre, Lucille: Belgian inventor talks by esophageal speech in four languages. *Cancer News, 20(2)*:22, 1966.

DiCarlo, Louis M., Amster, Walter W., and Herer, Gilbert R.: *Speech After Laryngectomy*. Syracuse, Syracuse U Pr, 1955.

Diedrich, William M., and Youngstrom, Karl A.: *Alaryngeal Speech*. Springfield, Thomas, 1972.

Doehler, Mary A.: *Esophageal Speech: A Manual for Teachers*. Boston, American Cancer Soc., 1953.

Duguay, Marshall: Preoperative ideas of speech after laryngectomy. *Arch Otolaryngol, 83(3)*:237, 1966.

Gardner, Warren H.: Problems of laryngectomees. *J Chronic Dis, 13(3)*:253, 1961.

Gardner, Warren H.: Rehabilitation after laryngectomy. *Public Health Nurs, 43(11)*:612, 1951.

Gardner, Warren H.: The Whistle technique in esophageal speech. *J Speech Hear Disord*, 27(2):187, 1962.

Gardner, Warren H., and Harris, Harold E.: Aids and devices for laryngectomees. *Arch Otolaryngol, 73(1)*:145, 1961.

Gargan, William: *Why Me: The Autobiography of William Gargan*. New York, Doubleday, 1969.

Gilmore, Stuart I.: Rehabilitation after laryngectomy. *Am J Nurs, 61(1)*:87, 1961.

Greene, James S.: Laryngectomy and its psychologic implications. *NY State J Med, 47(1)*:53, 1947.

Greene, James S.: Speech rehabilitation following laryngectomy. *Am J Nurs, 49(3)*:153, 1949.

Hodson, Cecil John, and Oswald, M. V. O.: *Speech Recovery after Total Laryngectomy*. Edinburgh, Livingstone, 1958.

Hudson, Atwood: An approach to the rehabilitation of the laryngectomized veteran. *Br J Dis Commun, 2(1)*:45, 1967.

Hyman, Melvin: An experimental study of artificial-larynx and esophageal speech. *J Speech Hear Disord, 20(3)*:291, 1955.

International Association of Laryngectomees: *Helping Words for the Laryngectomee*. New York, International Association of Laryngectomees, 1964.

International Association of Laryngectomees: *Rehabilitating Laryngectomees*. New York, International Association of Laryngectomees, 1960.

Johannessen, Jean V., and Foy, Audrey L.: Team effort in the rehabilitation of laryngectomy patients. *J Am Geriatr Soc, 12(11)*:1073, 1964.

King, Philip S. Fowlks, Everill W., and Peirson, George: Rehabilitation and adaptation of laryngectomy patients. *Am J Phys Med, 47(4)*:192, 1968.

King, Philip S., Marshall, Robert C., and Gunderson, Herbert E.: Management of the older laryngectomee. *Geriatrics, 26(4)*:112, 1971.

Lauder, Edmund: A laryngectomee's viewpoint on the intelligibility of esophageal speech. *J Speech Hear Disord, 34(4)*:355, 1969.

Lauder, Edmund: The role of the laryngectomee in post-laryngectomy voice instruction. *J Speech Hear Disord, 30(2)*:145, 1965.

Lauder, Edmund: *Self-Help for the Laryngectomee.* Edmund Lauder, 111115 Whisper Hollow, San Antonio, Texas, 1968.

Levin, Nathaniel M.: Recovering lost speech. *Rehabil Rec, 6(1)*:19, 1965.

Levin, Nathaniel M.: Speech rehabilitation after total removal of larynx. *JAMA, 149(14)*:1281, 1952.

Martin, Hayes: Rehabilitation of the laryngectomee. *Cancer, 16(7)*:823, 1963.

McCall, Julius W.: Preliminary voice training for laryngectomy. *Arch Otolaryngol, 38(1)*:10, 1943.

Miller, Maurice M.: The responsibility of the speech therapist to the laryngectomized patient. *Arch Otolaryngol, 70(2)*:211, 1959.

Monteiro, Lois: The patient had difficulty communicating. *Am J Nurs, 62(1)*:78, 1962.

Moses, Paul J.: Rehabilitation of the post-laryngectomized patient — the vocal therapist: Place and contribution to the rehabilitation program. *Ann Otol Rhinol Laryngol, 67(2)*:538, 1958.

Nelson, Charles R.: *Post-Laryngectomy Speech: You Can Speak Again!* New York, Funk and W, 1949.

O'Mara, Eloise: Still voice. *Reader's Digest, 70(5)*:65, 1957.

Pitkin, York N.: Factors affecting psychologic adjustment in the laryngectomized patient. *Arch Otolaryngol, 58(2)*:38, 1953.

Rovnick, Sydelle, and Sokolow, Esther: A case work experience with patients following loss of larynx. *Rehabil Lit, 26(5)*:135, 1965.

Sanchez-Salazar, Virginia, and Stark, Anne: The use of crisis intervention in the rehabilitation of laryngectomees. *J Speech Hear Disord, 37(3)*:323, 1972.

Schall, Leroy A.: Psychology of laryngectomized patients. *Arch Otolaryngol, 28*:581, 1938.

Shanks, James C.: Advantages in the use of esophageal speech by a laryngectomee. *Laryngoscope, 77(2)*:239, 1967.

Shryock, Harold: Speech without a larynx. *Hygeia, 25(10)*:752, 1947.

Snidecor, John C. (Ed.): *Speech Rehabilitation of the Laryngectomized,* 2nd ed. Springfield, Thomas, 1964.

Snidecor, John C., and Curry, E. Thayer: How effectively can the laryngectomee expect to speak? *Laryngoscope, 70(1)*:62, 1960.

Snidecor, John C., and Curry, E. Thayer: Temporal and pitch aspects of superior esophageal speech. *Ann Otol Rhinol Laryngol, 68(3)*:623, 1959.

Sykes, Eleanor M.: No time for silence. *Am J Nurs, 66(5)*:1040, 1966.

Wepman, Joseph M., MacGahan, John A., Rickard, Joseph C., and Shelton, Neil W.: The objective measurement of progressive esophageal speech development. *J Speech Hear Disord, 18(3)*:247, 1953.

Waldrop, William F., and Gould, Marie A.: *Your New Voice.* Chicago, American Cancer Society, 1969.

Chapter 9

SELECTED REHABILITATION PROFESSIONS

THE contents of this chapter could easily be expanded to include a dozen or more relevant professions such as dentistry, medicine, the ministry, nutrition, psychology, and social work. However, in order to pursue a rational system of delimitation, the author chose to discuss those professions most apt to deal directly with the patient on a daily basis in a rehabilitation (or maintenance) capacity.

NURSING

"The initials 'R.N.' and 'L.P.N.' mean to the world that you are in one of the most challenging, respected, exciting, and dynamic service professions or occupations." This quotation is from a "Health Career Facts" handout on nursing, available through the Health Careers Program, Madison, Wisconsin. Intending no malice toward this organization, the present author finds that this assessment could be easily paraphrased as follows: "You are in one of the most challenging, frustrating, turbulent, and demanding, yet least respected, service professions or occupations."

The author has repeatedly heard nurses say that professionally they do not know what they are. They are confused as to whether they are (or should be) bedside comforters, controllers of diets, drug administrators, temperature takers, surgical assistants, administrators, large hospital *ward bosses,* or any possible combination of these. Probably the one function on which there might be a reasonable degree of agreement is that of "meeting the immediate health care needs of the patient."

With this loosely defined function, one can consider the various areas of specialization, such as maternal and child, medical surgery, psychiatric, public health. Yes, the profession offers great challenge indeed!

To add to the confusion of the public and of health co-workers is the wide variety of educational backgrounds represented within any given nursing staff. Nursing education in this country uses a multitrack system leading to recognition as a RN (Registered Nurse). Further complicating the picture in recent years has been the introduction of such titles as *physician's assistant, pediatric nurse practitioner,* and a growing variety of others.

One means of preparation for nursing involves the successful completion of the requirements of a Bachelor of Science in Nursing (B.S.N.) which is nominally a four-year program. In reality, it can include additional summer sessions, or even a complete fifth year of study. The B.S.N., beginning with a liberal arts foundation, concentrates on the biomedical and social sciences. Most four-year programs include sixteen weeks of specialized preparation in each of the following: maternal and child health, medical surgery (chest and cardiac in particular), psychiatric nursing, and public health nursing.

Nurses holding the B.S.N. (as well as the comparatively smaller percentage which go on for graduate degrees) are the decision-makers — the members of the nursing staff responsible for critical inquiry resulting in plans of therapeutic action. These nurses independently plan nursing care for cases (outside the area of medicine), sharing responsibility for patient care with other members of the health team.

The nurses with a B.S.N. are also the only nurses prepared for the beginning level of public health nursing. Public health nurses are most interested in preventive aspects of their profession — particularly in the prevention of acute and chronic illness, and in early case finding. They treat the community at large, rather than working within a single institution.

Nursing education is also available through junior or community colleges. The Associate Degree (A.D.) is offered after completion of a two-year nursing program.

Another means of career preparation is through diploma programs. These are hospital based, rather than university- or college-based, programs requiring from twenty-four to thirty-six months to complete. Nurses prepared through hospital schools of nursing received a relatively small amount of training in biology and a tremendous amount of practical experience. In the United States there appears to be a trend developing in favor of the four-year baccalaureate nurse, and a phasing out of the diploma programs. Indeed, the American Nursing Association advanced such a goal in the 1965 ANA position paper.

Graduates of each of the three types of programs listed above (i.e. B.S.N., Associate Degree, and diploma program) are eligible to take state board examinations to become licensed as an RN. Upon granting of licensure, each nurse is entitled to the lifetime use of the term *Registered Nurse.* The capacity in which nurses are employed is highly dependent upon the employer and upon accessibility of nursing personnel. The baccalaureate nurse is the one most apt to rise to supervisory positions.

Much of a nurse's *know-how,* in addition to that arising from specialized instruction, comes through direct nursing experience, through hospital in-service education programs, and through updating skills and knowledge through university extension courses.

Two categories of paraprofessionals are Licensed Practical Nurses (L.P.N.'s) and Nursing Aides. L.P.N.'s must pass a board examination upon completion of a nine to twelve month post-high school course of studies. They work, at all times, under the specific direction of a Registered Nurse or a licensed physician. Nursing Aides (sometimes referred to as Nursing Assistants) are chiefly taught on-the-job. Their six-to-eight weeks of education involves some classroom instruction. They can offer simple care like bathing, temperature and pulse taking, and respiration observation. Their care is *nonjudgmental* in the sense that they are not made responsible for planning care.

Despite concern and disagreement about the roles they should play, nurses do accept as underlying duties their need to make total assessment — physically, mentally, emotionally, spiritually, and environmentally — and to start basic health care patterns, including referral and consultation. Since patient care practices include techniques appropriate to the newborn as well as to the dying aged (and all points along the womb-to-tomb continuum) the nurse necessarily interrelates closely with the professions of dentistry, medicine, dietetics, occupational therapy, physical therapy, speech pathology and audiology, psychology, social work, vocational rehabilitation, religion, etc.

The relative newness of the *total patient care* concept (or, continuity of patient care) involves working directly with the family and raises the question of "Who coordinates?" Should it be Social Service? Should it be the hospital's Director of Nursing? Many questions arise from the movement of patients in any direction in and out of the health care system. What continuity of care exists from home to hospital, from hospital to home, from hospital to extended care facilities, from hospital to nursing homes, etc.? How are the problems handled which arise out of special hearing and visual requirements? No matter how these questions are answered, it should appear obvious that any care which is truly patient-oriented cannot be oriented to any given service. Instead, the concept of teamwork must be advanced.

Nursing problems can involve vastly different dimensions dependent on the setting in which the nurse works. For example, in the hospital the patient fits the environment; in the home the nurse fits the patient's environment. In nursing homes there is a little of both.

In addition, concepts of rehabilitation differ between staffs of rehabilitation hospitals and those of acute hospitals (where initial therapies are begun). In our present era of changing care patterns, many acute hospitals — after life is saved and medical stability is achieved — discharge to nursing homes rather than to rehabilitation hospitals. Accordingly, there is pressure for nursing home staffs to become more familiar with rehabilitation, to pick up signs of potential which need to be assisted.

The nurse must continually resolve the extent of her unique contributions to such committees as the Bed Utilization Committee, the Patient Care Committee, the Record Review Committee, the Discharge Planning Committee. She is also expected to coordinate with such organizations as the local public health department and Visiting Nurse Association.

The truly successful nurse is said to be one who can adequately assess and minister to her patient's physical, emotional, and social needs. To do so requires communication with her patient despite whatever communication problems may exist.

Nurses, and most physicians, tend to be poorly prepared in the areas of speech and hearing. Although the nurse's education encompasses normal growth and development, such study is frequently restricted to motoric and emotional development. The nurse with a reasonably strong understanding of speech and language development is a relative rarity. Assessment of movement of the soft palate tends not to be within her range of competency. The average nurse has not been taught that anybody who has an eating problem has a speech problem (and frequently, vice versa). The hard-of-hearing patient may not receive the best care the nurse is capable of because of the nurse's lack of understanding of his communication impairment. What aspects of a speech pathologist's expertise should be conveyed to nurses? This question might most profitably be pursued in terms of "This will help *you* (the nurse) in caring for the patient" — not only, "This will help the patient." Such an approach might also minimize the reaction "What are *you* (the speech pathologist) doing with *our* (the nurses) patient?"

Ideally a typical nurse's "average day" would make productive use of every moment with the patient. Not only does the nurse discuss with the patient what is being done to him and why, but her activities extend out into the community — to the patient's family members, his doctor, his clergyman, his family, and to the Visiting Nurse Association, to nursing homes, etc., She interprets speech and hearing — like all the other patient needs — to all concerned. The nurse who understands best will best serve the patient's needs.

Rather than merely skimming in this chapter some of the speech, hearing, and perceptual problems with which nurses (and other health professionals) must contend, the reader is referred to the chapters dealing with additional problems of specialized populations, such as the hearing impaired and poststroke. The author's experience with rehabilitation leads to one inevitable conclusion: None of us, as rehabilitation specialists, can function effectively autonomously. The greatest values accrue to the patient who is approached by a staff completely imbued with the team approach. Ideal teamwork is not demonstrated by simply recording our professional observations in the patient's chart. (One Director of Nursing Services in a most distinguished and efficient hospital asked the author "Who do you honestly believe reads the charts?") Not only must the staff discuss the patient's needs and attitudes, but they need also to talk with the patient about what and how he is doing.

Other members of the staff, as well as family members, need to see the full array of the patient's problems. Each professional person has the responsibility to help all other members of the staff to see the problem as they see it. We all look through different filters.

Are there common problems that nursing, speech pathology, occupational therapy, and physical therapy can zero in on? Is there weakness of the respiratory and articulatory muscles? Can the muscle strengthening activities of physical therapy be coordinated with the speech needs of the patient?

What is the priority of the various problems faced?

Dependent on the given health or rehabilitation setting, such activities as chewing, sucking, and swallowing might be routinely developed by the nurse; in another setting, by the speech pathologist; by the occupation therapist in another. But we must know it *is* being done (if necessary) and by whom.

Is the occupational therapist working on feeding? If not, is the speech pathologist? If either or both of these two specialists are, we might appropriately ask whether, *in this institution,* ten minutes spent with the nurse might not be better than thirty minutes with the patient. Surely, the nurse would normally be the best bet to assure that speech (and its underlying more basic functions such as chewing, swallowing, sucking) is included in continuity of care!

If the speech pathologist routinely acquaints the other staff members with the patient's communication problems and how best to surmount them in the discharge of our duties, the other members of the rehabilitation team will seek advice from the speech pathologist on how they can further speech efforts while they are performing their own professional tasks. Simply to know they should attempt nothing — if that is the recommendation of the speech pathologist for a given patient at a given time — is helpful. The nurse and her aides can reasonably wonder what speech is appropriate while bathing the patient. Should they point to body parts, simultaneously naming them? Should they have the patient name parts? What speech activities should be *rewarded?*

Interprofessional awareness also minimizes problems by scheduling speech pathology at optimally relaxed times — *not* immediately following the enervating therapies.

What are our roles in working directly with the family? Is it possible that each separate professional is assuming that someone else is doing this? Surely it is mandatory that all members within the system understand that system and how it works.

Does the patient care plan reflect communication disabilities? Are these equally well understood by all pertinent staff members and by the family? During the predischarge home visit, in which the total home environment is assessed, do communication factors enter into the evaluation, or does such evaluation, terminate with consideration of physical and emotional factors only?

Successful communication is always a *two-way street.* The personalities of the communicators and the added communication breakdowns of the patient add to the difficulty. Virginia Stone (1969) believes there is a need for a different pacing of nursing care. *Expanded speech* has been found to facilitate appropriate responses. *Expanded speech* differs neither in loudness nor tone quality from normal speech, "it is just spread out more in time" (Panicucci, *et al.,* 1968). This does not mean that language structure is made more complex — it refers to slower presentation of all stimuli and allowing for extended periods of response time.

The communication system between the nurse's station and the patient's room is especially singled out (Stone, 1969) as requiring a nursing approach which makes optimal use of the patient's level of perception. This would include basic knowledge of pitch and loudness characteristics of speech, and utilizing one's voice accordingly, by pitching one's voice differently and avoiding shouting.

The 1970 *American Journal of Nursing* includes an article on "Standards for Geriatric Nursing Practice" (SEE Moses, 1970). The article presents an awesome list of nine standards, each accompanied by a rationale and examples. The communication aspects of many of these standards suggest the need for extensive interaction between members of nursing staffs and geriatric-oriented (and trained) speech pathologists. The article's recognition of cross-disciplinary problems is apparent, particularly in the standards dealing with speech deterioration, social interaction, sensory loss, nonverbal communication, and devices (including hearing aids).

However, is the nursing profession equally aware of the not-so-obvious deviations such as the peculiarities of communication deficits in left hemiplegia? Reference to this specific omission in the article should not be construed as negative criticism of what the article does expound. Indeed, the article is so impressive that it easily merits being made required reading for students of all the rehabilitation professions!

Members of the nursing staff spend more time with geriatric patients than any other professional group does. Accordingly, they must understand the factors which affect nurse-patient communication. It is probably impossible to overstate the force of nonverbal communication. The nurse's bedside manner — apart from the words she utters — will profoundly affect the degree to which her patient will attempt to communicate. Her own psychological needs will surely affect her ability to relate to her patients.

Recently a clinical specialist possessing a master's degree in nursing, told the author's class in the chronically ill and aged that one must not look at post-CVA's as stereotypes (i.e. left hemis, right hemis). She went on to say that "If you have them stereotyped, they sense this within a day." What is more basic is to understand "*a* person's problem" (rather than understanding *a ward* of aphasics).

This same nurse, employed by a rehabilitation hospital, posed the following questions: "How secure is the medical staff?" "Is it threatened by the nurses?" "Can they tolerate or respect a great amount of nurse responsibility?" It seems to the author that this same set of questions, directed at the speech pathologist, might effectively screen which rehabilitation programs incorporate optimal teamwork, which fall short.

At the same time, this nurse recognizes some built-in problems. Speech pathology, occupational therapy, and physical therapy services are usually accomplished on a one-to-one or one-to-two basis, seldom on a one-to-thirty basis as frequently experienced by nurses. Nurse's Assistants are not sufficiently knowledgable to carry out everything as well as nurses (who get orders from *every* specialty). Recognizing the basic difference in ratio of patient contact, the nurse suggests that other professionals keep coming back to educate the nurses. Nurses need more in-service education on alternative means of communication (nonverbal, for instance). We should all proceed on the assumption that if the other professionals have been turned off once, it is simply that they hit the nurse at saturation level.

OCCUPATIONAL THERAPY

Although the profession of occupational therapy is generally thought to have begun during the First World War, it probably dates from mineteenth century efforts to assist the mentally disturbed in asylums. It is believed that the momentum stemmed from nurses and physicians who thought purposeful activity would improve the physical and emotional stability of the patients.

While profession origin-tracing will probably remain speculative, it is easier to date the beginning of the training of occupational therapists in the United States to the year 1917 when the Surgeon General's concern led to a six-week training program to prepare *Reconstruction Aides* to serve injured soldiers in Army hospitals. Formal schools of occupational therapy were subsequently established, one of the first being that begun in 1918 at Milwaukee Downer College in Milwaukee, Wisconsin. This program was discontinued in 1967 after Milwaukee Downer College merged with and moved to Lawrence College in Appleton, Wisconsin. The Milwaukee Downer program is mentioned here, not only to recognize its pioneering role and its great merit for approximately half a century, but in recognition of the input of Downer's alumni in this text and because some of this book was written in the Downer building which formerly housed occupational therapy, and which subsequently became a part of the campus of the University of Wisconsin-Milwaukee.

The American Occupational Therapy Association (AOTA) defines occupational therapy as

> the art and science of directing man's participation in selected tasks to restore, reinforce and enhance performance, facilitate learning of those skills and functions essential for adaptation and productivity, diminish or correct pathology and to promote and maintain health. Reference to occupation in the title is in the context of man's goal-directed use of time, energy, interest and attention. Its fundamental concern is the development and maintenance of the capacity throughout the life span, to perform with satisfaction to self and others those tasks and roles essential to productive living and to the mastery of self and the environment (American Occupational Therapy Association, 1973).

A predecessor definition cited "any activity (be it social, creative, recreational, religious, etc.) medically prescribed and professionally supervised to increase, improve or maintain both physical and mental health" (Agatha Armstrong, in lecture, March 18, 1970).

In relation to any program for the aging, Diamond and Laurencelle specify the occupational therapist's role as "to provide, through individual support and planned activity, a sustained feeling of well-being, of usefulness, or recognition and respect and a continual reminder to the older person of his worth and meaning to society" (Diamond and Laurencelle, 1961).

Since the profession's early years, occupational therapists have stressed activity and creativity as part of the total person.

The work of an occupational therapist, according to Nancy Snyder (1970), focuses primarily on three major aspects: (1) *physical disabilities* (musculo-skeletal and/or neurological systems) and the need for independence in self-care, work, leisure, and play, with eventual return to society; (2) *perceptual-motor dysfunction* (developmental problems learning disabilities); and (3) *psychosocial dysfunction* (providing psychological support in helping the patient to adjust to disability).

Therapy is designed to help shorten hospital stay, minimize long-term effects, and effect independence. Specific approaches depend on the setting, the diagnosis, and the needs of the patient — seldom upon specificity of the referring physician's prescription which is apt to be couched in terminology as general as "Treat as indicated."

The registered occupational therapist will

> respond to a request for service whatsoever its course; the O.T.R. enters a case at his own professional discretion and on his own cognizance...(he) recognizes that the physician, duly licensed by the appropriate body to practice medicine and surgery, is the person who holds full responsibility for the medical management of a patient; (he) practices within the limits of competency and the supervisory pattern commensurate with his level of qualification...and treats, within the patient management plan, collaboratively with all others who care for the patient, and apprises the physician and appropriate supportive personnel of his findings and actions, all of which he documents in the legal medical record (American Occupational Therapy Association statement of June, 1969).

Therapeutic activities could include any of the major crafts of basketweaving, mosaics, jewelry making, metalwork, and printing. These activities would frequently be selected as part of the therapy in response to such specific physician prescriptions as "Increase strength in the right upper extremity," "Increase strength for crutch walking." Activities such as *sing along*, bowling, and the use of giant size (weighted) checkers might also be used.

Of particular importance is the occupational therapist's involvement in activities of daily living (ADL). These include transfer techniques, locomotion, dressing, eating, and personal hygiene. One-handed activities (frequently with the less dominant hand) include bathing, dressing, eating, personal grooming, and meal preparation.

The occupational therapist's evaluation is not only of the patient, but of the environment and its difficulties and hazards for the patient. For example, what problems does homemaking pose for the disabled woman in a wheelchair or walker? Are overhead slings required? What are the optimal locations for pots, pans, telephone, vacuum, stove controls, light switches, thermostats, water faucets? How can bedmaking and other household activities be achieved by hemiplegics, arthritics, and by individuals who must conserve their energies?

Experienced occupational therapists have a long history of using their imaginations (and carpentry skills) to modify environmental hazards for their patients. Their extensive use of adaptive equipment and *gadgets* — with its resultant tremendous physical and psychological benefits — offers a profitable learning situation for all other health and health related professionals. Use by members of the various professions of such items as blow bottles for maintaining respiration adequate for speech and mouth sticks for typing, should help us all to recognize legitimate areas of professional overlap — to view a situation not as a specific profession's problem, but as a patient problem.

In addition to the role of direct treatment, occupational therapists might be expected to participate in testing, evaluation, research, administration, community programs, vocational programs, education, and consultation.

Registered Occupational Therapists (OTR's) work in a variety of settings including hospitals (orthotics, pediatrics, geriatrics), rehabilitation centers, mental institutions, orthopedic schools, teaching institutions, public health agencies, home services, long-term care facilities (TB, mental health, and V.A. hospitals, curative workshops, and rehabilitation hospitals), and nursing homes. They work with children, the deaf, the blind, the physically handicapped, the emotionally and mentally disturbed, the geriatric population, and with the following orthopedic or neurological disabilities: CVA, spinal cord lesions, arthritis, amputations, cerebral palsy, brain damage, CNS damage-disorders, parkinsonism, muscular dystrophy, multiple sclerosis, fractures, and other orthopedic conditions.

At present there are approximately fifty approved baccalaureate programs in the United States preparing occupational therapists, or OTR's (Registered Occupational Therapists). Registration is accomplished through the American Occupational Therapy Association (AOTA) upon completion of an accredited program, required field work, and successful passing of the examination for admission to the National Registry of the AOTA. Under present regulations, once the National Registry examinations are passed, the person remains registered as long as he maintains membership in the American Occupational Therapy Association. He is eligible to practice anywhere in the world where he can be understood.

Baccalaureate degrees in occupational therapy are comprised of two years of liberal arts study, followed by specialization in the last two years. These curricula include *physical and behavioral sciences* (including anatomy, neuroanatomy, physiology, neurophysiology, neurology, chemistry, physics (applied and abnormal), psychology, sociology, kinesiology) *clinical subjects* (including general medicine, surgery, orthopedics, psychiatry), *manual and creative skills* (including leatherwork, weaving, ceramics, woodworking, metalwork, basket weaving, printing), and *activities of daily living*.

The post-B.S. year's internship is in general medicine, pediatrics, psychiatry, and orthopedics.

Some universities prepare occupational therapists whose undergraduate major was in one of the sciences. They offer postbachelor's course work of approximately twenty months' duration, divided between academic and clinical work.

Master's degrees are also offered by a limited number of universities.

Obviously the types of persons thus qualified are not to be confused with subprofessionals whose activiti es have helped give rise to the highly undesirable label, *play ladies*. The various recreational or activity directors, while performing admirable tasks in various settings, are frequently associated with occupational therapy departments, hence creating confusion in the public mind as to the qualifications and competencies of OTR's.

The Certified Occupational Therapy Assistant (COTA) is a

person trained to perform treatment under the supervision of an OTR. This specialist is being trained under the sanction of the national organization — the AOTA.

OTR's and COTA's who work with the aged adapt their activities in recognition of the factors which limit or hamper learning in old age. Allen Pincus lists these factors as "(1) insufficient response time, (2) stress or arousal of anxiety in the learning situation, (3) lack of motivation of the subject, (4) difficulty in discriminating between environmental stimuli, and (5) psycho-motor deficits in responding to such stimuli" (Pincus, 1968).

The occupational therapy profession has greatly expanded since World War II, particularly in Veterans Administration hospitals where it was historically divided into music therapy, recreation therapy, and industrial arts. Prior to the establishment of V.A. departments of speech pathology, the physician's prescription to the OT frequently read "This person should learn to verbalize." It is easy to understand the OT's potential involvement in speech activities, since patients make limited progress in ADL if unable to hear, see, or talk. If communication with the patient is impossible, the OT can only work at *passive* activities.

Anyone relating to people in a therapeutic setting must establish satisfactory communication with the patients or residents. This does not mean that everyone should become a speech pathologist. However, there is a certain amount of basic communication information, the mastery of which will help any professional to function more effectively *within his own professional role(s)*.

By the nature of their patient goals and activities, occupational therapists should be particularly well suited to integrate into their program appropriate speech and language activities as outlined by the local speech pathologist. For example, see the 1965 article listed in this chapter's References by McGeachy.

Likewise, the speech pathologist must realize that occupational therapy provides many opportunities for verbal directions. It provides an opportunity to carry on simple, direct, and (hopefully) meaningful conversation with the patient. The occupational therapist can increase his effectiveness by utilizing one-word commands. He can be encouraged to watch, wait, and listen. But in addition to cooperation between the speech clinician and the occupational therapist, there is also a need for cooperation between all the therapists, the patient, and staff. Observation and interaction are mandatory.

The occupational therapist is particularly valued by the speech pathologist in assisting to devise alternative means of communication when needed. Perhaps speech pathologists have done too little along nonverbal communication lines. For example, a picture board portraying specific wants or activities can make a considerable difference in the life of one unable to read. Similarly a word board, with appropriate nouns, verbs, etc., could be utilized with other patients. Even an alphabet board may serve some patients, e.g. the nonintelligible speaker with the use of a good hand. (See the chapter on stroke for a further discussion of nonverbal communication).

The physically limited might appreciate charts (with words or pictures of toilet, eating, razor, comb, sleeping, wheelchair, etc.) with adaptations for head movement controls or foot-controlled pointers or light beams. Electronic aids, such as devised to meet the needs of cerebral palsied children (see Holmlund and Kavanagh, 1967), incorporate sucking and blowing to adjust radio, TV, and temperature controls.

Geriatric patients suffer reduced sensory input not only due to malfunction and disuse, but also from psychological retreat from the environment. Patient care plans, therefore, should include training in sensory discrimination. They might involve increased auditory and visual stimulation (large print and sound amplication, for example), as well as efforts to reinforce the patient's contacts with reality.

Occupational therapists also are expected to cope with the problems of remotivation. Senior citizens need to feel that they belong to a group, they need to experience self-determination and independent action. Janice Klein, an OTR, and Joseph Lidington, a COTA, set forth the following therapeutic objectives of a physical, occupational and recreational program:

a. Socialization and restoration of self-respect.

b. Fostering of interpersonal relationships (self-confidence).

c. Stimulation of interest and prevention of mental deterioration.

d. Motivation and maintenance of emotional well-being.

e. Role definition — learning how to participate — male and female.

f. Helping physical well-being and functioning — maintaining and improving physical status.

g. Releasing of tension and stimulating desire to renew old interests and develop new ones (Klein and Lidington, 1968).

Two activities which occupational therapists have found greatly beneficial as geriatric treatment tools are choral reading (see Powell, 1961) and group reading (Johnston, 1965). Ms. Johnston reports on thirteen sessions devoted to reading the book *Episode* (about a stroke patient). She reports that good group feeling developed early in the sessions; the residents began to discuss openly and understand better their disabilities, and they shared their experiences of frustrations. Such activities can bring about the *cohesiveness* necessary for giving patients a feeling of security and to counteract the feelings of loneliness so common in institutions.

The use of readings, along with discussions of "the world we live in", constitute much of the basis for *remotivation therapy* — a psychosocial treatment program that assists in the rehabilitation of those who have *given up*.

The occupational therapist can help other professionals by observing (1) how the patient communicates his needs, (2) how he attracts the therapist's attention, (3) how the patient relies on gestures and facial expressions, and (4) how successful the patient's speech attempts are. The occupational therapist — as well as the physical therapist and the speech pathologist — recognizes the need to know what is going on throughout the patient's day, not simply "He's *my* patient until noon." He must know whether his patient slept well, just had a sedative, or is just plain sleepy. One can only learn these details by communicating with the other professionals and aides.

PHYSICAL THERAPY

The purpose of physical therapy is to correct, alleviate, or prevent human physical or mental disability following stroke or injury, and to intervene and prevent the progression of disease.

Patients appear as a result of sport injuries (fractures, sprains, strains, nerve injuries, torsion, and spinal cord injuries), industrial injuries (amputations, laceration of tendons and nerve, burns, fractures, back strains — especially herniated discs), auto injuries (burns, spinal cord problems, skull fracture, brain damage), and home accidents (with equipment used for mowing lawns, tree trimming, snow removal, home carpentry, etc.). Illness, disease, and aging also provide patients, particularly those suffering strokes, parkinsonism, multiple sclerosis, cerebral palsy, etc. The aging, in particular, present problems such as hip fractures, arthritis, arteriosclerosis, and respiratory diseases, including emphysema.

Direct services to patients include the treatment of illness and injury by physical and chemical means such as light, heat (conductive, infrared, deep), water, electricity, ultrasound, as well as massage and therapeutic exercise. These techniques are used to improve circulation, restore motion, relieve pain, strengthen muscles, and correct deformities, thereby assisting in the restoration of physical and economic independence.

An RPT (Registered Physical Therapist) is trained to evaluate the following: ADL (activities of daily living), self-care, gait, strength, joint measurement, posture, nerves, elasticity, coordination. RPT's are also qualified to plan the following: prevention, maintenance, restoration, consulation, and research. In recent times, many physical therapists have extended their activities into schools (helping to screen for scoliosis), into the therapeutic use of ultrasound, and into obtaining EMG's (electromyograms).

In their services to patients of all ages, physical therapists assist in relieving pain, shortening hospital stays, and improving the long-range outlook for activity.

Needless to say, such goals cannot be achieved in a professional vacuum. Instead, they require close cooperation between such various members of the health team as physicians, nurses, occupational therapists, prosthetists or orthotists, inhalation therapists, psychologists, psychiatrists, social workers, vocational counselors, the patient's family, and the patient himself. Indeed, without the first-mentioned team member — the physician — there would be no physical therapy, since physical therapy is done only upon *prescription* by a physician.

The specificity of the prescription depends greatly on the working relationship of the given physician and physical therapist. It may simply read "Employ appropriate treatment to accomplish the desired results." The prescription may specify resistive exercise, diathermy, etc. It might be stated in terms of a goal, i.e. "Ambulatory with aid of a walker." The technique and modality choice may be left to the discretion of the physical therapist (who subsequently discusses the appropriate care plan with the doctor). It may indicate precautions, or list things which are contraindicated. The more the treatment minutae are spelled out, the more the physical therapist becomes a mere technician. The referral might also specifically indicate the desirability or necessity for teaching the patients and their families about the care of equipment, etc.

Although the role of *direct treatment* is that most readily apparent in the functioning of most physical therapists, it must be recognized that educative and research roles can also play a large part in the professional activities of a given physical therapist. New therapists need to be taught. Home health aids need to be trained. Consultation needs must be met.

The ideal use of physical therapists in direct treatment is probably achieved in settings offering truly patient-centered care and patient-centered staffings. Joint patient assessment and evaluation involving mutual interprofessional effort frequently produces interdisciplinary in-service education in preventive and restorative techniques, resulting in agency personnel better trained in disability prevention and long-term care. This succeeds best in an atmosphere of open communication and interprofessional trust. The recognition of overlapping skills leads to less concern about exclusive rehabilitation *territories* such as ADL and ambulation. Formerly, the patient and his care were fragmented. Since all involved professionals have impact on the same patient, they ought to share their patient insights. The roles of each professional must modify to the extent that the services become patient- rather than profession-centered.

To recapitulate, then, the major functions of a physical therapist are as follows:

1. EVALUATION: to evaluate muscle strength and cardiovascular status, and to test for neurological damage and respiratory problems under the prescription of a legally licensed physician.

2. PLANNING: to outline a treatment program as a result of his evaluation and present a list of recommendations to the physician.

3. APPLICATION: to implement his therapeutic procedures, applying psychological and sociological principles (i.e. treating the whole patient, including the family).

4. INSTRUCTION: to teach the nonprofessional workers functioning in nursing homes, as well as the family and family substitutes.

5. COMMUNICATION: to cooperate with other health professionals in a team approach.

6. EDUCATION: to participate in public education.

What are the educational requirements for practicing as a physical therapist? There are presently three main types of training programs. All three require the bachelor's degree as a minimum. The traditional bachelor's program, with a major in physical therapy, is found chiefly in major universities with medical schools. This program can be completed in four years. Supervised clinical practice is required. It is customary for the last semester, or a postdegree semester, to be spent in obtaining clinical experience. There are slightly over fifty such programs in the United States. These programs stress the humanities and social sciences, while concentrating heavily on the sciences, including anatomy, biology, chemistry, pathology, physics, physiology, and kinesiology (joints, muscles, and bones in action).

A twelve to sixteen month *certificate* program is available in some training institutions to applicants who already possess a bachelor's degree in one of the basic sciences. The third type of program for students with the requisite background culminates in a master's degree. This degree is frequently taken in anatomy, physiology, vocational counseling, or public health.

As of the time this chapter was written, all states but one had instituted licensing procedures. Typically such licensure requires membership in the American Physical Therapy Association, graduation from a school approved by both the American Physical Therapy Association and the American Medical Association, and satisfactory completion of written and/or oral examinations. Licensure qualifies the person to work as a RPT. Reciprocity is fairly general between states.

In the past decade, two types of physical therapy subprofessionals have come into being. PTA's (Physical Therapy Assistants) are the products of Associate Degree (two-year) programs. These individuals can work only under the supervision of RPT'S. They cannot do evaluations, muscle testing, or electrodiagnosis; they cannot initiate treatment programs.

A second type of subprofessional is the P.T. Aide. The Aide completes an on-the-job training program given by a RPT. The time duration for such a program is not specified by the states, and could vary greatly in terms of hours. An aide cannot administer treatment unless the RPT is physically present.

Another classification is that of *corrective therapist.* These specialists arose from the Medical Corps during World War II. They were trained on-the-job by RPT's for gait training and resistant muscle training. Their function is similar to that of aides. They can neither assess nor plan a program of treatment. They work in army or V.A. hospitals.

Physical therapists work in a wide variety of professional environments. They work in hospitals and in specialized institutions for children, veterans, and people with orthopedic conditions or chronic diseases. They work in medical clinics in industry. They work in rehabilitation centers. They work in private practice. They work as teachers and as researchers.

To better understand the limitations (or expanding horizons) of services offered by a given RPT, it is best to analyze the local elements which affect patient care. These would include the community finances, the program, the personnel, the agency, and the type of patient.

SPEECH PATHOLOGY AND AUDIOLOGY

The profession of speech pathology and audiology got its start in America under the auspices of public education, rather than through medicine, as was the case in Europe. It would appear from available records that the cities of Chicago and Detroit are the chief contenders for the credit of first employing a specialist in the public schools to deal exclusively with speech disorders (Pagel Paden, 1970). The year 1910 marks the initiation of school assistance to youngsters whose speech was judged to be abnormal or inferior.*

The first Ph.D. granted to a person trained specifically to work "experimentally and clinically with speech and hearing disorders" (see Johnson, 1955) was awarded in 1924. The recipient of this initial degree was Lee Edward Travis; the university granting the degree was the University of Iowa.

At the time of Dr. Travis' doctoral studies there was a heady intellectual atmosphere in Iowa City, spurred on in particular by psychologist Carl Emil Seashore. Dr. Seashore, who was to serve as chairman of the Department of Psychology and Dean of the Graduate School, was particularly adept in getting representatives of various professions or disciplines to discuss areas of overlap. It was in these areas that he believed the most significant discoveries would occur. The discipline of speech pathology was born in large part as a result of his probing the minds of members of the medical school faculty, psychology department, physics department, etc.

Lee Travis, in his doctoral studies, was free to sample the teaching in any classroom of the university, remaining as long as he felt he could benefit. It was this type of intellectual inquiry that hastened the birth of speech pathology as a discipline at the University of Iowa.

Similarly, others were intrigued with the possibility of measuring hearing levels and hearing loss electronically. The people primarily interested in this activity ultimately became known as *audiologists*. It is difficult to ascertain from the records

---

*This statement excludes teachers of the deaf who were working with the speech and language of deaf youngsters prior to this time.

extant exactly how early individuals were involved in similar activities at the University of Wisconsin in Madison and at Northwestern University, the other major pioneers in this field.

The origins of the American Speech and Hearing Association (ASHA) are also clouded in uncertainty. It is said that the forerunner of the ASHA had its inception in the Iowa City home of Lee Edward Travis or in the living room of Dr. Robert West at the time he was teaching in Madison or in the trophy room of New York City's Hotel McAlpin (Pagel Paden, 1970). This meeting (or meetings) was (were) held in 1925 — a year after Lee Edward Travis concluded his formal doctoral studies at Iowa.

Because the major demand for remedial services arose within the public schools of this country, many of the early academic training programs began in state teacher's colleges. Most of these early programs clustered in the midwest. The early programs usually appeared within schools of education or in speech departments within the College of Arts and Science, or Letters and Science, or whatever name was deemed appropriate (or was currently fashionable) in a given institution. From the start, most training programs drew upon the resources of many departments such as speech, education, psychology, physics, anatomy, neuroanatomy, and sociology. Succeeding years saw an increasing need for specialists in speech and hearing to work in hospital or rehabilitation settings, frequently with more severely- and multiply-involved cases.

Specifics of academic training programs — whether preparing people to work in educational or in medical environments — were never standardized nationally. However, what is standardized is a minimal number of credit hours in specified areas of study, as well as a minimal number of clock hours of clinical experience with cases.

During the early developmental period, a rash of identifying labels were applied to the products of such educational programs. These included *speech correctionist, speech therapist, speech clinician, speech pathologist,* and even *speech teacher*. In some cases a term was written into state laws dealing with the certification of these school specialists. At present, there is no nationwide standardization or agreement upon a particular term, but the American Speech and Hearing Association is using and recommending the term *speech pathologist* in dealing with representatives of state and federal governments (see Johnson, 1968, for extensive comments on terminology).

The recent proliferation of knowledge, vastly expanded concepts dealing with maladaptive behaviors, and greater sophistication in sociological and anthropological concepts helped the profession to view its baccalaureate degree studies as insufficient. By 1970 it was necessary to possess a master's degree in order to become certified as clinically competent by the American Speech and Hearing Association. Additional requirements are to subscribe to the organization's code of ethics, to complete a year of supervised professional experience after completion of the master's degree, and to pass a written national examination.

This raising of academic standards was accomplished with certain grandfathering provisions, so it is possible to encounter individuals recognized as clinically competent who do not possess the master's degree.

Perhaps of greater confusion is the fact that clinical competence is certified in what superficially appear to be two seemingly separate and disparate areas: (1) speech pathology and (2) audiology. However, speech and hearing professionals, through their organization the American Speech and Hearing Association, reconfirmed in the ASHA's 1969 Legislative Council that "Speech pathology and audiology form areas of a single profession" (ASHA Legislative Council, 1970). Unfortunately the profession was not able to agree upon a shorter, less ambiguous generic term.

The use of the word *certification* can also bear some clarification. Certification by the American Speech and Hearing Association is not binding on all speech and hearing clinicians. Through the years another type of certification has existed — that offered by state departments of public instruction. Minimal training experiences for such state certification vary widely, although a good many states have accepted the ASHA standards as minimal. A person certified to practice speech pathology in a public school *may not* have met requirements as stringent as those required for ASHA certification.

The move to license speech pathologists and audiologists has gained considerable momentum in recent years. As of the time these words were written, approximately one third of all the states had formally adopted licensure. If most of the remaining states follow suit, the problems arising out of certification will undoubtedly vanish.

Expectations of a practitioner of this profession can be gleaned from a recent article on the philosophy and operation of the national examinations in speech pathology and audiology. This article, in describing the national examinations, states that

> The speech pathology test covers basic and applied knowledge for clinical practice. Basic areas may include descriptive, physiologic, acoustic, and perceptual phonetics; anatomy and physiology; instrumentation and interpretation of research; language, including normal development, psycholinquistics, and semantics; and psychology, including learning, child development, adjustment, and intelligence and personality testing. Applied knowledge covers disorders of communication associated with neuropathologies, including such categories as cerebral palsy, dysarthria, aphasia, and brain injured children; orofacial pathologies, including cleft palate; laryngopathologies and laryngectomy; psychological aspects of difficulties in articulation, voice, rhythm, and language, including such categories as stuttering, autism, mental retardation, and delayed development; and basic audiology. Evaluation and treatment of the various disorders are included. Ethics or professional practice are also covered (Perkins, *et al.*, 1970).

With respect to the testing of audiology applicants, the authors indicate that

> The major content areas covered by the audiology test are psychoacoustics; anatomy and physiology, including physiological acoustics; auditory impairment, including symptomatology, etiology, and pathology; evaluative techniques; habilitation and rehabilitation, including amplification, speech reading, auditory training, speech conservation, and education of the deaf. Other areas covered by the test are acoustics, including properties of the signal and medium,

measurement, and scales; instrumentation, including calibration techniques, testing equipment, and technical aspects of hearing aids; developmental and geriatric aspects of audiology; research applications and statistics; speech science and speech pathology, including basic knowledge of normal mechanisms and their relation to audition; hearing conser-vation programs; and the administration and organization of a speech and hearing facility (Perkins, *et al.*, 1970).

Specifically, what is it that a speech and hearing clinician does when he works professionally? As already noted it is possible to be certified in two different areas. First, let us consider the individual whose clinical competency has been certified in audiology. The type of work which involves most audiologists in this country is that of hearing assessment, hearing aid assessment, and hearing conservation. By hearing assessment is meant the testing of an individual's hearing to ascertain not only his residual hearing acuity, but also his ability to discriminate one sound from another. In the event that a hearing aid is potentially suggested by pure tone and speech reception tests, the audiologist will progress to hearing aid evaluation. He would attempt to ascertain whether any type of aid improves hearing sufficiently to merit the required expenditure on the part of the client. His findings, in conjunction with those of an otologist, are also used to suggest the site of lesion in the case of central types of hearing loss.

A certain percentage of all audiologists also engage in audiological research, including study of the normal hearing process. The audiologist may also, dependent upon his training and inclination, work with the total communication process of the hard-of-hearing person by supplying training in speech reading.

Let us now consider the person who is clinically certified in speech pathology. Traditionally this person has worked with four main types of communication problems: articulation, voice, rhythm, and language. How might these be encountered in individuals with communication impairments?

No matter how we define *articulation,* we refer to the manner in which speech sounds are produced. For instance, if I talk about a "wed wabbit wunning down the woad," I am in essence demonstrating an articulation error which we can further categorize as a /w/ for /r/ substitution. Because of the close relationship between articulation disorders and intelligibility (i.e. the degree to which speech is understandable), articulation problems have been considered more or less paramount within our school systems. If a child cannot speak in such a way that he can be understood, the schools justifiably are very concerned. However, except in severe problems of articulation, it is questionable as to whether this type of problem should consume the majority of the school speech pathologist's case load.

Fluency disorders tend to attract more unfavorable attention than slightly distorted, single-sound articulation problems. The two major types of fluency disruptions are the seeming inability to initiate a sound (commonly referred to as a person's inability to *break through,* or inability to *get the word out)* and the seeming inability to prevent repetition of a sound or syllable that has already been produced (i.e. reiteration, such as "g-g-g-g-g-go").

The third main grouping of communication disorders with which the speech pathologist works is called *voice* disorders. By this term we refer to peculiarities in tone quality arising from abnormal phonation or abnormal resonating of the phonated tone. Appropriate voice depends on both the anatomical and physiological integrity of the series of chambers above the vocal folds (e.g. the throat, mouth, and nose) as well as the integrity of the vocal folds themselves. In the absence of such integrities we are called upon to deal with such problems as breathy voice, excessively nasal voice, and hoarse voice quality.

The fourth type of communication disorder that speech pathologists have been traditionally concerned with is that of *language*. From the very beginning of our profession that person called a speech correctionist or speech pathologist has been called upon to deal with language problems — particularly of the adult aphasic. This term's referents will not be belabored in this chapter. The interested reader can pursue them in the chapter on stroke.

The upsurge of interest in language during the past two decades has been not only with respect to the brain-damaged adult demonstrating aphasic speech, but also with the youngster who has an inadequate vocabulary for his age, or who has never apparently acquired adequate syntactic skills. This inability has frequently been misinterpreted as reflecting a low mental capacity or a hearing deficiency.

Concomitant with the development of this grave concern over impairments in the development of language was the attention given to differences noticed between different cultural subgroups. We have progressed from talking about the *culturally disadvantaged* to the *culturally distinctive,* or the *culturally different.* A great amount of activity has been generated by speech pathologists interested in specializing with these types of communication differences.

In summary, the speech pathologist is concerned with problems of articulation, voice, rhythm, and language. No matter what subpopulation of individuals we are concerned with — be it aphasic, cleft palate, cerebral palsied, multiple sclerotic, Parkinson — the communication problems fall into one or more of these categories, and can be aggravated by concomitant problems of hearing, intelligence, social deprivation, aging, etc.

Dependent on his preferred professional specialty, a speech pathologist may choose to work in elementary and secondary schools, university and college clinics, in hospitals (acute, children's, rehabilitation, and V.A.), rehabilitation centers, and in private practice.

One's responsibilities may be direct case care (diagnosis and therapy — including counseling), consultation, research, teaching, administration, or any given combination of these activities.

Many speech pathologists' initial patient encounters are at bedside where family members may or may not be present. Clients are brought to us in rehabilitation centers or as outpatients to hospitals where we may or may not meet family members. The patients are seen in our small, materials-cluttered clinical-office rooms where they come and leave on the hour and the half-hour in tightly regimented traffic patterns. It would seem that such regimentation is largely due to pressures for our service to break even financially, or even to make money to bail out less financially successful departments in our nonprofit institution.

Patients seeking our help must enter this regimentation and conform to it.

Patients with catastrophic health problems (especially poststroke) present family and community problems. Family stability is at stake. Patient-peer interactions must be interpreted. Patient problems such as limited memory span, suicidal tendencies, epileptic attacks, changes in sexual functioning, alterations in role, or adaptation to paralysis need attention. The patient and his family must cope with medical, psychological, communication, social, nutritional, moral and financial problems. Many of these problems cry out not only for rehabilitation of the patient, but of the family as well.

How is family counseling to be improved? How will better public education on these matters come about? It is exceedingly frustrating to many speech pathologists that such counseling and educative services in most treatment centers are not normally revenue bearing.

If the nonspeech pathologist reader of this book has the benefit of working with a speech clinician well trained and knowledgable in serving the chronically ill and aged, you undoubtedly are working with a clinician who is crusading for better team approaches in patient care, and for TV-monitored clinical facilities which simulate the average home's living room, bedroom, bathroom, and kitchen — environments in which better therapeutic and counseling activities can be pursued with the patient *and* with members of the patient's family.

REFERENCES

American Occupational Therapy Association: Description of Occupational Therapy, Oct. 29, 1973.

American Occupational Therapy Association: Statement on Occupational Therapy Referral, June 1969.

American Speech and Hearing Association Legislative Council: Report of the legislative council, ASHA. *ASHA, 12(4)*:186, 1970.

Diamond, Mary V., and Laurencelle, Patricia: The role of the occupational therapist in the care of the geriatric patient. *Am J Occup Ther, 15(4)*:139, 1961.

Holmlund, B. A., and Kavanagh, R. N.: Communication aids for the handicapped. *Am J Occup Ther, 21(6)*:357, 1967.

Johnson, Wendell: Communicology? *ASHA, 10(2)*:43, 1968.

Johnson, Wendell: The time, the place, and the problem. In Johnson, Wendell, and Leutenegger, Ralph R. (Eds.): *Stuttering in Children and Adults: Thirty Years of Research at the University of Iowa.* Minneapolis, University of Minnesota Press, 1955.

Johnston, Nancy: Group reading as a treatment tool with geriatrics. *Am J Occup Ther, 19(4)*:192, 1965.

Klein, Janice and Lidington, Joseph: PT, OT and RT. *Professional Nurs Home, 10(11)*:31, 1968.

McGeachy, D. J.: The role of the occupational therapist in the rehabilitation of speech. *Can J Occup Ther, 23*:53, 1965.

Moses, Dorothy V., *et al:* Standards for geriatric nursing practice. *Am J Nurs, 70(9)*:1894, 1970.

Panicucci, Carol L., Paul, Penelope B., Symonds, Jean M., and Tambellini, Josephine L.: Expanded speech and self-pacing in communication with the aged. *American Nurses' Association 1968 Dallas Clinical Sessions.* New York, Century-Crofts, Meredith Corporation, 1968.

Pagel Paden, Elaine: *A History of the American speech and Hearing Association, 1925-1958.* Washington, American Speech and Hearing Association, 1970.

Perkins, William, Shelton, Ralph, Studebaker, Gerald, and Goldstein, Robert: The national examinations in speech pathology and audiology: Philosophy and operation. *ASHA, 12(4)*:175, 1970.

Pincus, Allen: New findings on learning in old age: Implications for occupational therapy. *Am J Occup Ther, 22(4)*:300, 1968.

Powell, Evelyn Jane Dressler: Choral reading as an activity. *Am J Occup Ther, 15(2)*:67, 1961.

Snyder, Nancy: Perspectives on a rehabilitation theme: occupational therapy. Paper read at "Perspectives on a Rehabilitation Theme: Interdisciplinry Function in Patient Care" — a Continuing Education Short Course, Indiana Regional Medical Program, Nashville, Indiana, Sept. 25, 1970.

Stone, Virginia: Give the older person time. *Am J Nurs, 69(10)*:2124, 1969.

ADDITIONAL READING LIST

Nursing

Anonymous: Financial Aids: Nursing careers. *Health Careers Program* (P.O. Box 289, Madison, WI, 53701), 1969.

Baltz, Florence L., and Reardon, Ross A.: Medicare and nursing homes. *Nurs Outlook, 14(6)*:55, 1966.

Bender, Ruth E.: Communicating with the deaf. *Am J Nurs, 66(4)*:757, 1966.

Burchett, Dorothy E.: Factors affecting nurse-patient interaction in a geriatric setting. *ANA Regional Clinical Conferences, 1967: Philadelphia / Kansas*

City. New York, Appleton, 1968.

Burt, Margaret M.: Perceptual deficits in hemiplegia. *Am J Nurs, 70(5)*:1026, 1970.

Calnan, Mary E.: In-service in nursing homes. *Nurs Outlook, 16(2)*:43, 1968.

Coye, Dorothy H.: Programmed instruction for staff education. *Am J Nurs, 69(2)*:325, 1969.

Evangela, Sister M.: Love provides the reason. *Nurs Outlook, 17(6)*:39, 1969.

Fleer, Paul F.: The role of therapists on the home health agency team. *Health, 18(2)*:9, 1967.

Hentgen, Janice H.: Dressing activities for disabled persons. *Nurs Clin North Am, 1(3)*:483, 1966.

Isler, Charlotte: New specialty: Nursing in the extended-care facility. *RN, 31(6)*:30, 1968.

Jones, Wendell E., and Kramer, Charles H.: Creating a therapeutic language atmosphere. *Professional Nurs Home, 9(9)*:46, 1967.

Juzwiak, Marijo: This speech/hearing rehab center benefits both patients and RN's *RN, 27(1)*:38, 1964.

Kalson, Leon: The therapy of discussion. *Geriatrics, 20(5)*:397, 1965.

Large, Helen, Tuthill, Joseph E., Kennedy, F. Bryan, and Pozen, Thomas J.: In the first stroke intensive care unit. *Am J Nurs, 69(1)*:76, 1969.

Lefevre, Margaret C.: Speech therapy for the geriatric patient. *Geriatrics, 12(12)*:691, 1957.

Luterman, David M., Welsh, Oliver L., and Melrose, Jay: Responses of aged males to time-altered speech stimuli. *J Speech Hear Res, 9(2)*:226, 1966.

Miller, Michael B.: Synthesis of a therapeutic community for the aged ill. *Geriatrics, 21(8)*:151, 1966.

Mitchell, Joyce: Communication in the geriatric unit I. *Nurs Times, 65(14)*:423, 1969.

Mitchell, Joyce: Communication in the geriatric unit II. *Nurs Times, 65(15)*:465, 1969.

Mitchell, Joyce: Communication in the geriatric unit III. *Nurs Times, 65(16)*:495, 1969.

Mitchell, Joyce: Disorders of communication in the older patient. *Gerontol Clin (Basel), 6*:331, 1964.

Mitchell, Joyce: Speech and language impairment in the older patient: Some problems in management. *Geriatrics, 13(7)*:467, 1958.

Rolnick, Michael I.: Speech pathology services in a home-health agency: The Visiting Nurse Association of Detroit. *ASHA, 11(10)*:462, 1969.

Spencer, Gwendolyn E.: The cerebral vascular accident patient. *Nurs Outlook, 8(6)*:326, 1960.

Spencer, Marian G.: The aged patient in a chronic disease hospital. *Nurs Outlook, 10(9)*:594, 1962.

U.S. Department of Health, Education and Welfare: *Elementary Rehabilitation Nursing Care* (Public Health Service Publ. No. 1436). Washington, U.S. Government Printing Off, 1966.

Weihofen, Henry, and Usdin, Gene L.: Who is competent to make a will? *MH, 54(1)*:37, 1970.

Occupational Therapy

Feallock, Barbara: Communication for the non verbal individual. *Am J Occup Ther, 12(2)*:60, 1958.

Jackson, Barbara N.: The occupational therapist as consultant to the aged. *Am J Occup Ther, 24(8)*:572, 1970.

Jennings, Frank J.: Language: Bridge or barrier. *Am J Occup Thr, 13(4)*:190, 1959.

Johnson, Jerry, and Smith, Margaret: Changing concepts of occupational therapy in a community rehabilitation center. *Am J Occup Ther, 20(6)*:267, 1966.

Miller, John, and Carpenter, Carolyn: Electronics for communication. *Am J Occup Ther, 18(1)*:20, 1964.

Ness, Agnes Dick: Positive and negative techniques to employ and avoid with the auditory handicapped. *Am J Occup Ther, 7(1)*:16, 1953.

Norton, Carolyn, and Towne, Carol C.: Occupational therapy for aphasic patients. *Am J Occup Ther, 22(6)*506, 1968.

Olsen, Janice Z., and May, Bella J.: Family education: Necessary adjunct to total stroke rehabilitation. *Am J Occup Ther, 20(2)*:88, 1966.

Richman, Leona: Sensory training for geriatric patients. *Am J Occup Ther, 23(3)*:254, 1969.

Roberts, Dean W.: Occupational therapy for the chronically ill. *Am J Occup Ther, 14(4)*:171, 1960.

Schoening, Herbert A., and Iversen, Iver A.: Numerical scoring of self-care status: a study of the Kenny self-care evaluation. *Arch Phys Med Rehabil, 49(4)*:221, 1968.

Wisconsin State Division of Health: *Bed Activities, Transfers and Walking for the Hemiplegic Patient*. Wisconsin State Division of Health. Undated, but of 1970 origin.

Wisconsin State Division of Health: *Bed Positioning and Maintenance of Joint Motion for the Hemiplegic Patient*. Wisconsin State Division of Health, 1970.

Physical Therapy

Boone, Daniel R.: Relationship of progress in speech therapy to progress in physical therapy. *Arch Phys Med Rehabil, 42(1)*:30, 1961.

Davis, Joan Lynne: Teamwork in speech and physical therapy. Phys Ther Rev, 32(9):452, 1952.

Egland, George O.: Physical therapy, occupational therapy, and speech therapy.

J Am phys Ther Assoc, 46(10):1116, 1966.
Elson, Mildred O.: The geriatric patient. *J Am Phys Ther, 42(2)*:101, 1962.
Hurwitz, L. J.: Sensory defects in hemiplegia. *Physiotherapy, 52(10)*:338, 1966.
Morrison, Letty W.: Physiotherapy in the geriatric assessment unit. *Physiotherapy, 52(8)*:269, 1966.

Speech Pathology and Audiology

American Speech and Hearing Association: code of ethics of the American Speech and Hearing Association, 1974. *ASHA, 16(6)*331, 1974.
American Speech and Hearing Association: Requirements for the certificates of clinical competence. *ASHA, 15(2)*:77, 1973.

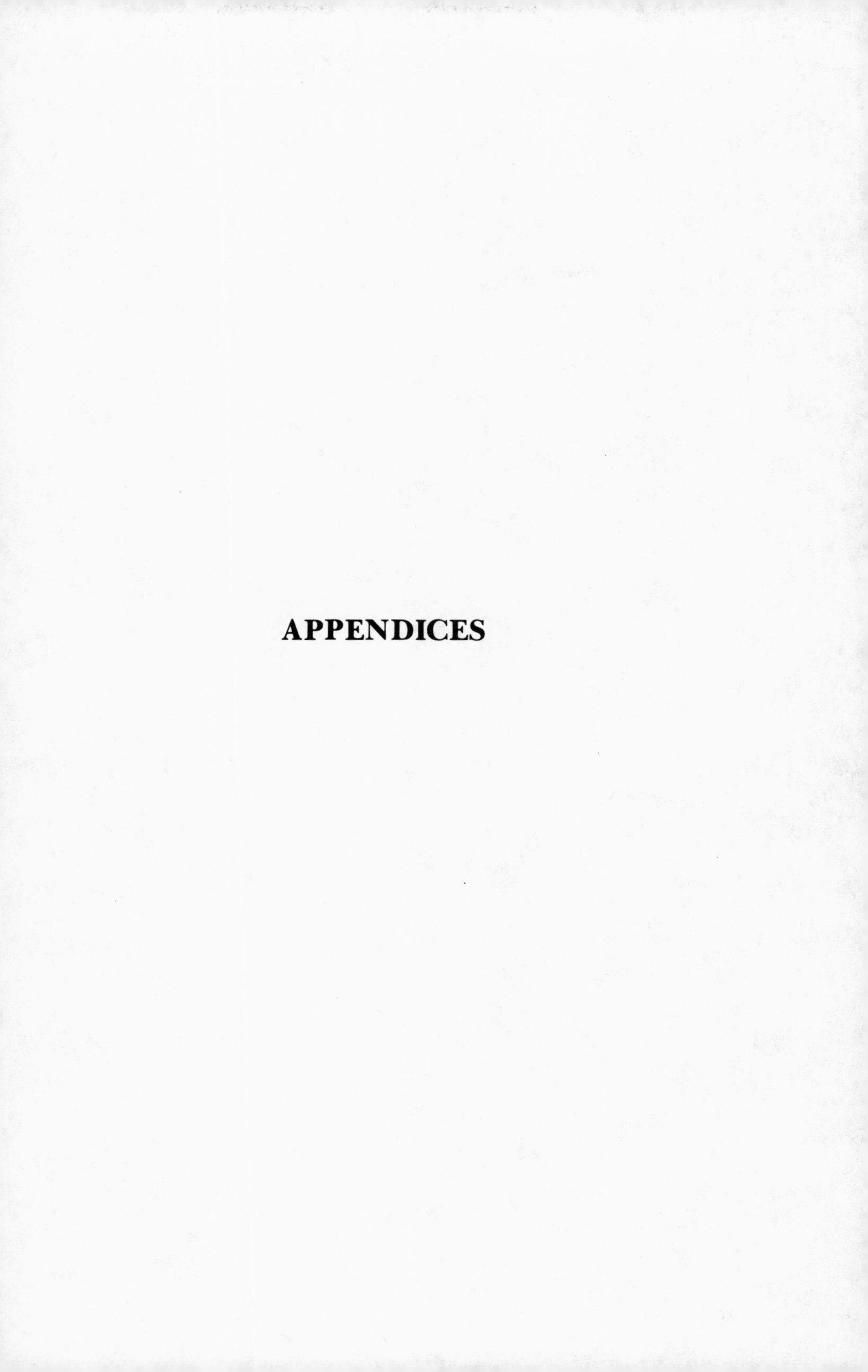

APPENDICES

APPENDIX A

AMERICAN ENGLISH CONSONANT SOUNDS

(Presented in symbols of the International Phonetic Alphabet (I.P.A.)

	Stop	*Fricative*	*Nasal*	*Lateral*	*Glide*	*Affricate*
Bilabial	p b		m		w; hw	
Labiodental		f v				
(Lingua) dental		θ ð				
(Lingua) alveolar	t d	s z	n	l	l; r	
(Lingua) palatal		ʃ ʒ			j; r	tʃ dʒ
(Lingua) velar	k g		ŋ			
Glottal		h				

KEY:

In each pair of sounds, the first of the pair is voiceless (VL), the second voiced (V). Sounds separated by a semicolon are independent of each other and not V–VL pairs.

The [r] appears in two places to indicate two alternative tongue positionings (place of articulation).

The [l] appears in two places to indicate it is *always* a lateral, sometimes a glide.

[θ] – "th" as in thin	[ʒ] – "zh" as in leisure	[tʃ] – "ch" as in church
[ð] – "th" as in then	[ŋ] – "ng" as in ring	[dʒ] – "dz" as in judge
[ʃ] – "sh" as in shoe	[j] – "y" as in yes	

Square brackets are used to set off phonetic symbols from orthographic script.

APPENDIX B

A Survey of Aphasia Diagnostic Tests

Language Modalities Test for Aphasia (LMTA)

Joseph M. Wepman and Lyle V. Jones
Education-Industry Service
1225 E. 60th Street
Chicago, Illinois 60637

The earliest test to be considered is the Language Modalities Test for Aphasia (LMTA) copyrighted in 1961 by Joseph M. Wepman and Lyle V. Jones. The initial twenty-four items by themselves constitute a screening test for aphasia. Wepman and Jones suggest that the degree of success or failure on these twenty-four items will determine whether or not it is profitable to proceed with the entire test. The items in this screening test include verbal naming, spelling, repeating, and arithmetic solutions. They also include copying two geometric figures, writing words, and pointing (matching forms, pictures and words) as a result of an oral request. The items are scored as acceptably completed or as failed. In other words, there are twenty-four plus-minus items.

The total LMTA (1) includes the screening items just noted; (2) explores spoken and written skills; (3) requires matching responses which are scored on a plus-minus basis; (4) screens oral and graphic responses which are scored on a six-point scale; in addition to (5) including a short *tell-a-story*. The tester is encouraged to indicate the case's ability to correct his own errors. The test manual recommends recording various types of maladaptive behavior observed such as stuttering, dyslalia, euphoria, and fatigue. The relative lack of specificity in administration procedures would appear to have an adverse effect on reliability.

The LMTA is intended to do the following, according to its designers: it "seeks responses in speech and writing" (to standard visual and auditory stimuli); "it tests comprehension of language symbols as well as the ability to imitate them along both common input modalities"; and "it deals briefly with form recognition, arithmetic ability, spelling, and articulation. It provides separate information about the adequacy of symbolic and non-symbolic language behavior... It provides a measure of (the patient's) ability to use syntax as well as vocabulary" (Wepman and Jones, 1961).

This test accomplishes in a telescopic manner a sampling of each of the skills the constructors claim are being tested. The test constructors infer that the test will yield an *impression* of classification category. This includes pragmatic, semantic, syntactic, jargon, and global aphasia, as well as agnosia and apraxia. The administrative manual is of little help in indicating how to arrive at these classifications based on the results of the testing. The briefest of hints is afforded by short citations of speech judged to be typical of these classifications, as well as three case summaries — one of pragmatic, one semantic, and one syntactic aphasia.

Administration of the LMTA requires auditory stimuli by the examiner, as well as the use of two 35 mm filmstrips, a filmstrip viewer, a spiral bound subject's response booklet, a spiral bound examiner's record booklet, a scoring summary (and history) sheet, as well as a manual for administering, plus an instruction manual. Apart from the costs involved, the potential user may need to consider the need for spiral bound booklets for each administration, plus the ability to comfortably use a filmstrip viewer. The test has the advantage of having two comparable forms. "The usual time for administering one complete form is approximately one hour. However, for many Subjects more time will be required" (Wepman and Jones, 1961). It is unclear how therapy suggestions are to be derived from the completed test, or how to use the test as a prognostic device.

Minnesota Test for Differential Diagnosis of Aphasia (MTDDA)

Hildred Schuell
The Psychological Corporation

304 E. 45th Street
New York, New York 10017

Another major test which ahs had widespread use is Hildred Schuell's 1965 form of the Minnesota Test for Differential Diagnosis of Aphasia (MTDDA). The claim made for this test is that it provides for exhaustive testing in several major areas of possible language disturbances. Because of its length, it is usually necessary to spread the administration of this test over several clinical sessions. The test presents a sampling of auditory disturbances, visual and reading disturbances, speech and language disturbances, visuomotor and writing disturbances, as well as disturbances in numerical relations and arithmetic processes. Each of these various areas or subtests are scaled according to difficulty, hence a baseline and a ceiling can be derived for each subtest. A summary of test scores presents a fairly concise grouping of the revealed disturbances.

It is assumed that the administrator of this test will move from this summary of test scores to a seven-fold classification of the type of language problem based on pattern of impairment. A rather general prognostic expectation (e.g. *excellent, limited*) is available for each of the seven classifications.

As in the LMTA, the MTDDA is similarly limited in not clearly indicating appropriate therapeutic practices. On the other hand, the relationship of therapy rationale to test findings is less tenuous when augmented by the recommendations contained in the book *Aphasia in Adults,* written by Hildred Schuell, James J. Jenkins, and Edward Jimenez-Pabon. An abbreviated form ("A Short Examination for Aphasia"), intended as a screening device, is described in the 1957 issue of the journal *Neurology.*

Materials required to administer the MTDDA include standardized score booklets, an administrative manual, and two spiral bound sets of cards. In addition, the clinician must furnish some common objects not included with the test materials.

In summation, it would appear that both the LMTA and the MTDDA yield reasonable samplings along a continuum of communication function. It is assumed that the skilled tester can (1) classify the type of aphasia involved, and (2) derive therapy suggestions from the language deficiencies revealed.

The Sklar Aphasia Scale (SAS)

Maurice Sklar
Western Psychological Services
Box 775
Beverly Hills, California

The Sklar Aphasia Scale (SAS), was published in 1966 by Maurice Sklar. This screening device requires a sequence of tasks at fairly basic levels in each of four modalities: auditory decoding, visual decoding, oral encoding, and graphic encoding. Despite its reported high correlations of .97 with the MTDDA and .92 with the 1954 "Examining for Aphasia" by Jon Eisenson, the manual's lack of specificity on administration instructions can only serve to depress the test's (and tester's) reliability. This scale yields an impairment score which, after a simple conversion to percent of impairment, is roughly translated into a prognosis, i.e. *favorable, uncertain, unfavorable.*

Length of time needed to administer this test is said to be less than an hour. Its use is inappropriate in assessing minimal language deficits.

The Porch Index of Communicative Ability (PICA)

Bruce Porch
Consulting Psychologists Press
577 College Avenue
Palo Alto, California 94306

The Porch Index of Communicative Ability (PICA) appeared in 1967 and is now available in a 1971 revision. In the years since its first appearance, Dr. Bruce Porch's test has generally become known as the PICA. The PICA, like the LMTA, usually requires approximately one hour to complete. Administration of the test involves obtaining 180 descriptions of how the patient performs in a situation testing various communication skills. Involved are eight subtests requiring gestural responses, four verbal tests, and six tests of writing and copying ability. These are achieved with two standard placements of materials, said materials consisting of two of each of the following: cigarette, comb, fork, key, knife, matches, pencil, pen, quarter, and toothbrush. These items are provided in an attaché case, along with a spiral bound test format booklet and three sets of stimulus cards. Also supplied are score sheets and profile sheets, in addition to a manual covering administration and scoring, as well as one which discusses underlying theory and the test's development. A third manual, presenting more detailed information on interpretation, was said to be *forthcoming* at the time this chapter was written. The test kit supplies all materials necessary except a ball point pen, a watch or clock (for timing responses), and a large, clean desk blotter.

Perhaps the major divergence of the PICA from the LMTA and the MTDDA is its use of a multidimensional scoring technique. This technique enables indicating the accuracy, completeness, efficiency, and promptness with which the patient makes his responses. It also involves recording the amount of information the subject needs before he can make an appropriate response (responsiveness). These five aspects are encompassed within the scoring process which requires the tester to assign a number from 1 to 16 for every task required of the person being tested. The critical factor involved in the usefulness of this test is the reliability of the tester. Dr. Porch claims that a training period of at least forty hours is minimal for acquiring proficiency in testing. The author's personal reaction is to underscore the word *minimal* in Porch's statement.

The procedures which must be followed after the administration of the test are time-consuming. However, the numerical test scores can be converted into an overall mean response level and mean response levels for each modality, as well as into visual profiles which help to diagnose, to chart the progress of cases, and to make six-month prognoses with a reasonable degree of accuracy. Once the tester becomes skillful at plotting profiles and interpreting them, he should be able to discern quickly between each of these five different types of problems: (1) aphasia without complications, (2) aphasia with verbal formulation or expression problems, (3) aphasia complicated by illiteracy, (4) patients with bilateral brain damage, and (5) aberrant patterns in which the communicative disorder is not aphasia. The latter would include such things as motor function problems and malingering.

Not only do the test profiles, when plotted over time, reveal when the patient has reached maximum benefit from his treatment, but they also yield precise suggestions to the clinician on the types of tasks with which to begin therapy. Testing locates the point on the continuum at which the patient is functioning. Treatment is "directed at those tasks and skills which are adjacent to the most difficult tasks at which the patient has complete success" (Porch, 1971).

Although many clinicians will feel that the frustrations and time involved in becoming a proficient PICA tester are well worth the effort, the PICA cannot be looked to as the definitive answer to *all* adult poststroke language testing. For example, it is of limited usefulness for cases demonstrating a minimal degree of severity, and for individuals with right hemisphere damage.

The Appraisal of Language Disturbance (ALD)

Lon L. Emerick
University Press
Northern Michigan University
Marquette, Michigan

A more recently copyrighted language diagnostic test to be used with adults is the ALD (the Appraisal of Language Disturbance) published by Lon L. Emerick in 1971. Dr. Emerick is interested in inventorying a patient's abilities with respect to various modalities of input and output, and central integrating processes. Accordingly, the subtests in his test are designated as follows: aural to oral, aural to visual, aural to gesture, aural to graphic, gesture to visual, visual to gesture, visual to oral, and visual to graphic, as well as central language comprehension, and a tenth set of *related factors* which include arithmetic tasks. The test samples approximately 250 language tasks. Unlike the LMTA, the MTDDA, and the PICA, this test has not been validated in the usual research manner.

The ALD claims to describe the nature and extent of language impairment in acute aphasic patients, but it does not attempt to place the aphasic into any classification system. Its devisor wishes to avoid "hardening of the categories" (Emerick, 1971). Instead of classifying, a summary-profile is derived from the patient's responses, utilizing a five-point scale of correctness of response.

The ALD comes in an attaché case which includes the test manual, display cards, card series, color shapes, *hand* puzzle, and eight-page test protocol booklets. The tester must supply some common objects not included with the test materials.

Dr. Emerick claims that his test "provides a detailed description of a patient's ability to receive and express messages by means of the various modalities of input and output"; it serves as "a basis for implementing speech rehabilitation" (by selecting the best avenues of approach); "it provides information which permits the clinician to offer intelligent advice and counseling to the patient's family, his nurses and others concerned with the aphasic's care"; "it provides the clinician with information for making a prognosis for the patient with regard to language recovery"; and "it provides a frame of reference for measuring the efficacy of language therapy" (Emerick, 1971). The first claim is probably more justified and apparent than the remaining ones.

The Boston Diagnostic Aphasia Examination (BDAE)

Harold Goodglass and Edith Kaplan
Lea and Febiger
600 Washington Square
Philadelphia, Pennsylvania 19106

In 1972 Harold Goodglass and Edith Kaplan published the Boston Diagnostic Aphasia Examination (BDAE). They advanced three possible purposes or aims of aphasia testing: "(1) diagnosis of presence and type of aphasic syndrome, leading to inferences concerning cerebral localization; (2) measurement of the level of performance over a wide range, for both initial determination and detection of change over time; (3) comprehensive assessment of the assets and liabilities of the patient in all language areas as a guide to therapy" (Goodglass and Kaplan, 1972). In the judgment advanced by the test's constructors, the test's satisfaction of all three of these purposes makes it "maximally useful to the neurologist, the psychologist, the speech pathologist and the speech therapist" (Goodglass and Kaplan, 1972).

Goodglass and Kaplan provide speech profile ratings and Z-score profiles for five major aphasic syndromes: Broca's aphasia, Wernicke's aphasia, anomic aphasia, conduction aphasia, and transcortical sensory aphasia. They further describe — but without supplying illustrative test patterns — these additional syndromes: transcortical motor aphasia, alexia with agraphia, aphemia, pure word-deafness, pure alexia, pure agraphia, and the following callosal disconnection syndromes — unilateral tactile aphasia, unilateral agraphia and apraxia, and hemioptic aphasia.

The test is divided into five subtests: (1) Conversational and Expository Speech, (2) Auditory Comprehension, (3) Oral Expression, (4) Understanding Written Language, and (5) Writing. Additional language and nonlanguage tests, not incorporated into the aphasia battery, "cover an exploration of psycholinguistic factors in auditory comprehension and in expression, exploration of disorders of repetition, study of the sparing of comprehension of whole body movement commands and screening for hemispheric disconnection symptoms" (Goodglass and Kaplan, 1972).

The test can be used to evaluate the following areas of deficit: articulation, verbal fluency, word-finding ability, verbal repetition, seriatim speech, grammar and syntax, paraphasia, auditory comprehension, reading, and writing.

The test's designers discuss the limitations as those "inherent in any aphasia test. The materials and procedures provided by the test merely serve as convenient aids for sampling relevant performances of the patient. The scores do not objectively and automatically classify the patient nor point to the optimum approach to therapy" (Goodglass and Kaplan, 1972). Goodglass and Kaplan proceed further to note that usefulness of interpretations rests upon the experience of the examiner, and that "the case illustrations will serve as a guide but not as a source of cookbook formulas for diagnosis" (Goodglass and Kaplan, 1972). The chapter on *Statistical Background* notes that "Test-retest data have not been obtained with this instrument" (Goodglass and Kaplan, 1972). No claims are made for prognostic usage.

Administration of this test requires a test form, a set of stimulus cards, and the basic manual which describes the evolution of the test and supplies supplementary tests, in addition to setting forth administration procedures and interpretation (test patterns of major aphasic syndromes). Administration time is said to vary from one to four hours.

Functional Communication Profile (FCP)

Martha Taylor
Institute of Rehabilitation Medicine
New York University Medical Center
(Rehabilitation Monograph No. 42).

The next two tests to be discussed appear superficially to bear a strong resemblance to each other. This apparent resemblance is minimized upon closer scrutiny. Perhaps the basic difference between Martha Taylor's Functional Communication Profile (FCP) and the Wisconsin Division of Health's Communication Status Chart (CSC) is that the former was intended for use only by experienced clinicians "having access to hundreds of aphasic patients in any given year" (Taylor, 1963). Martha Taylor, now Mrs. Sarno, cautions that "the form may have little validity when used by inexperienced personnel having only intermittent contact with aphasics or access to small case loads" (Taylor, 1963).

Possibly this qualification arose out of Martha Sarno's definition of *normal* as being equal to the patient's estimated premorbid communication effectiveness in terms of accuracy, rate, and mode of performance, as well as latency of response. Varying, therefore, with the patient's premorbid educational, social, and intellectual level, such rating puts "a severe burden upon the clinician to develop his own stable reference framework" (Taylor, 1963).*

Mrs. Sarno's test utilizes an eight-point rating scale and a conversion chart which yields an overall percentage score as well as five subscores which convert to percentages, enabling one to tell from one retest to the next the specific area in which the patient has improved (or regressed). The three major areas she labels *speaking, understanding,* and *reading.* A fourth area called *movement* has to do with aspects of both verbal and nonverbal communication, while the fifth category — *other* — is a miscellaneous category requiring the patient to write his name, and evaluating his time orientation, his copying ability, his ability to write from dictation, his skill in handling money, his ability to write in lieu of speech, and his calculation ability. In view of the heterogeneous aspect of this category, the interpretation of its mean score is less meaningful than the other four areas evaluated.

Sarno notes that the patient's responses elicited for this profile should be based on informal interaction with the patient, and not the result of performance rating in response to clinically presented language tasks. Hence, no standardized materials are required, and no claims are made for prognostic usage. Estimates of administration time are inappropriate since the FCP is not a traditional standardized test.

Communication Status Chart (CSC)

Wisconsin Division of Health
Madison, Wisconsin 53701

Information for completing the Wisconsin Division of

---

*It may be of considerable interest for the reader to be aware of the conclusions drawn at the Kenny Rehabilitation Institute upon terminating three reliability and two validity studies of the FCP. They concluded that "Even though the raters knew nothing about the patient's premorbid language level, they agreed that a particular *FCP* overall score was representative of a unique level of general communicative adequacy. This implies that a premorbid baseline is not essential to functional measurement as had been suggested by the author of the *FCP*.... The analyses of the data suggest that the *FCP* is measuring functional communication ability with reference to a standard index of communicative adequacy and not in reference to the patient's premorbid language ability" (Thomas P. Anderson, Norman Bourestrom, and Frederick R. Greenberg, *Rehabilitation Predictors in Completed Stroke* [Minneapolis, Kenney Rehabilitation Institute, 1970]).

Health's Communication Status Chart (CSC) is derived from testing, reading the patient's medical records, as well as by observing and questioning both the family and patient. It is the intent of the Wisconsin test that this screening be accomplished by personnel other than certified speech pathologists. It is contended that anyone possessed of an average level of intelligence and serious interest in the patient's welfare should be able to use this assessment instrument. The CSC assesses the patient's vision, his hearing, his dentition, chewing and swallowing skills, as well as the following language and language-related activities: verbal expression, general comprehension, writing, reading comprehension, and arithmetic.

The philosophy underlying the use of the CSC is that an awareness of the patient's ability in these various skills and an awareness of visual, auditory, and dental problems should be of help to each person relating with the patient in a care or rehabilitation capacity. The completed chart should tell such personnel the reason for wearing glasses (for distance or close work) and the apparent effectiveness of their glasses; the amount of time that a hearing aid is worn (always, usually, occasionally, never) and its seeming ability to help the patient's hearing; the condition of the natural teeth as well as the presence and frequency of use of dentures; plus various skills necessary for sucking, chewing, and swallowing.

In the language skills section of this screening test the person completing the screening indicates the effectiveness of verbal expression — whether it is restricted to sounds, words, phrases, or meaningful sentences, as well as lower level attempts such as babbling, mimicking speech, and inappropriate speech. The area devoted to general comprehension indicates the patient's ability to recognize common objects, to follow simple commands, and to indicate appropriate answers to simple questions and to a paragraph. Again, on a lower level it records whether the patient is aware of environmental sounds, the appropriateness of yes-no answers, and his ability to identify parts of the body. Similarly the skills of writing and reading and arithmetic are assessed. Part of the arithmetic task is to ascertain the patient's skills in handling money, in recognizing time, and his ability to write three- or four-digit numbers. These tasks are in addition to the normal arithmetic tasks of addition, subtraction, multiplication, and division.

The CSC does not yield a score *per se* since it is a screening, not a diagnostic, test. All items represent an accomplishment or a deficit. Within certain areas the tasks appear in a sequence of difficulty enabling the person who reviews the sheet to determine the level at which the patient is performing. It should be further noted that there is no time limit stipulated for completing this screening chart. It is simply a helpful aid to all involved in patient care and rehabilitation.

Consultants of the Wisconsin Division of Health, who use this assessment tool for in-service training in nursing homes and homes for the aged, report that staffs, once they can effectively complete the screening chart, report its considerable usefulness in helping to better understand the varying care problems of their residents or patients.

Necessary materials to be used in completing various sections of the test are available in loose-leaf form, protected by plastic, through the Section of Facilities Assistance, in the Bureau of Health Facilities, Division of Health, State of Wisconsin. The person completing this assessment must also supply a small number of common objects.

The Token Test for Receptive Disturbances in Aphasia (TT)

E. DeRenzi and L. A. Vignolo

The Token Test (TT) evolved from efforts to create a test useful in discovering receptive disturbances not readily apparent in the usual clinical examination or in conversation with the patient. The test's designers — E. DeRenzi and L. A. Vignolo — were interested in creating a test which could be administered in a short time, which would require no special apparatus or printed materials, which would be easy for the tester to administer, and which would require of those tested the least intellectual level coupled with considerable linguistic difficulty.

The resultant test, utilizing twenty *tokens* in two sizes, two shapes, and five colors, appears to meet the criteria set forth by its designers. The test proceeds with progressively more complex instructions to manipulate (touch, move, or pick up) the tokens. Of special value is "the lack of redundancy of the message transmitted to the patient and the necessity, which this entails, of grasping its significance from the semantic value of every single word he hears" (DeRenzi and Vignolo, 1962).

A validity study by B. Orgass and K. Poeck (1966) found the test to be highly discriminatory for individuals over fifteen years of age, regardless of the clinical type of aphasia. They located a cutoff point for differentiating the normal from the pathological, i.e. eleven errors or less.

The test, originally designed for Italian subjects, remains unstandardized in English at the time of this writing. However, there appears to be a great deal of interest in the United States in the test and its clinical use. Of particular promise is the Revised Token Test (RTT) designed by Malcolm R. McNeil and Thomas E. Prescott. The RTT utilizes a PICA-type fifteen-point scoring system. McNeil and Prescott, at the time this was written, were readying their normative data for publication.

Other Tests

No discussion of contemporary aphasia tests — despite a self-imposed limitation to *recent* tests — should fail to acknowledge the tremendous debt owed to Jon Eisenson for his pioneering test (1946) "Examining for Aphasia and Related Disturbances" (The Psychological Corporation, 304 East 45th Street, New York, New York 10017).

Although not specifically designed for use with aphasics, the following tests have proven helpful in affording various aphasiologists with additional client insights: Lloyd M. Dunn's 1959 *Peabody Picture Vocabulary Test* (American Guidance Service, Inc., 720 Washington Avenue S.E., Minneapolis, Minnesota, 55414); J. C. Raven's 1958 *Progressive Matrices* (New York, Psychological Corporation); the 1948 *Full-Range Picture Vocabulary Test* by Robert B. Ammons and H. S. Ammons (Missoula, Montana, Psychological Test Specialists); the 1959

Leiter International Performance Scale, (Santa Barbara, State College Press); and J. M. Wepman's 1958 *Auditory Discrimination Test* (Chicago, J. M. Wepman).

REFERENCES

DeRenzi, E., and Vignolo, L. A.: The token test: A sensitive test to detect receptive disturbances in aphasics. *Brain, 85*:665, 1962.

Emerick, Lon L.: *ALD — Manual for Appraisal of Language Disturbance.* Marquette, University Press, Northern Michigan University, 1971.

Goodglass, Harold, and Kaplan, Edith: *The Assessment of Aphasia and Related Disorders.* Philadelphia, Lea & Febiger, 1972.

Orgass, B., and Poeck, K.: Clinical validation of a new test for aphasia: an experimental study on the Token Test. *Cortex, 2*:222, 1966.

Porch, Bruce E.: Porch Index of Communicative Ability, Vol. 2, Revised edition. *Administration, Scoring, and Interpretation.* Palo Alto, Consulting Psychologists Press, 1971.

Schuell, Hildred: A short examination for aphasia. *Neurology, 7*:625, 1957.

Schuell, Hildred: A re-evaluation of the short examination for aphasia. In Sarno, Martha Taylor (Ed.): *Aphasia — Selected Readings.* New York, Appleton, 1972.

Schuell, Hildred: *Differential Diagnosis of Aphasia with the Minnesota Test.* Minneapolis, U of Minn Pr, 1965.

Schuell, Hildred, Jenkins, James J., and Jimenez-Pabon, Edward: *Aphasia in Adults.* New York, Hoeber, 1964.

Taylor, M. L.: *Functional Communication Profile.* New York, Institute of Rehabilitation Medicine, 1963.

Taylor, Martha L.: A measurement of functional communication in aphasia. *Arch Phys Med Rehabil, 46*:101-107, 1965.

Wepman, Joseph M., and Jones, Lyle V.: *Studies in Aphasia: An Approach to Testing.* Chicago, Education-Industry Service, 1225 East 60th Street, 60637, 1961.

APPENDIX C

References for Families of Adult Aphasics

Author	*Title*	*Date*	*Source*
Agranowitz, Aleen, and McKeown, Milfred R.	*Aphasia Handbook for Adults and Children*	1964	Chas. C Thomas, Publ. 301-327 E. Lawrence Ave Springfield, Illinois 62703
American Heart Association (Joseph M. Wepman, Consultant)	*Aphasia and the Family*	1969	American Heart Assoc. 44 E. 23rd Street New York, New York 10010
Boone, Daniel R.	*An Adult Has Aphasia*	1965	Interstate Printers and Publishers, Inc. 19-27 N. Jackson St. Danville, Illinois 61832
*Buck, McKenzie	*Dysphasia: Professional Guidance for Family and Patient*	1968	Prentice-Hall, Inc. Englewood Cliffs, New Jersey 07632
*Cameron, Constance C.	*A Different Drum*	1973	Prentice-Hall, Inc. Englewood Cliffs, New Jersey 07632
Cohen, Lillian Kay	*Communication Problems After a Stroke*	1971	Kenny Rehabilitation Institute 1800 Chicago Ave. Minneapolis, Minnesota 55404
Farrell, Barry	*Pat and Roald*	1969	Random House Inc. 201 E. 50th Street New York, New York 10022
Griffith, Valerie Eaton	*A Stroke in the Family: A Manual of Home Therapy*	1970	Dell Publishing Co., Inc. 750 Third Avenue New York, New York 10017
Halpern, Harvey	*Adult Aphasia*	1972	Bobbs, Merrill Co., Inc. Indianapolis, Indiana

*Hodgins, Eric	*Episode: Report On the Accident Inside My Skull*	1964	Atheneum Publishers 122 E. 42nd Street New York, New York 10017
Horwitz, Betty	*An Open Letter to the Family of an Adult Patient with Aphasia*	1962	*Rehabilitation Literature 23(5)*:141, May, 1962 (Reprint available from Nat'l Soc for Crippled Children and Adults, 2023 W. Ogden Ave. Chicago, Illinois
Houchin, Thomas D., and DeLano, Phyllis Janes	*How to Help Adults With Aphasia*	1964	Public Affairs Press 419 New Jersey Ave SE Washington, D.C.
Keith, Robert L.	*Speech and Language Rehabilitation: A Workbook for the Neurologically Impaired*	1972	Interstate Printers and Publishers, Inc. 19-27 N. Jackson St Danville, Illinois 61832
Knox, David R.	*Portrait of Aphasia*	1971	Wayne State University Press Detroit, Michigan
Longerich, Mary Coates	*Manual for the Aphasic Patient*	1958	Macmillan Publ Co., Inc. 866 Third Ave New York, New York 10022
Longerich, Mary Coates, and Bordeaux, Jean	*Aphasia Therapeutics*	1954	Macmillan Publ Co., Inc. 866 Third Ave New York, New York 10022
*McBride, Carmen	*Silent Victory*	1969	Nelson-Hall Co., Publ. 325 W. Jackson Blvd Chicago, Illinois 60606
*Moss, Claude S.	*Recovery with Aphasia: The Aftermath of My Stroke*	1972	University of Illinois Press Urbana, Illinois
Peterson, Jean C., and Olsen, Ann P.	*Language Problems After a Stroke: A Guide for Communication*	1965	Kenny Rehabilitation Inst. Minneapolis, Minnesota

*Ritchie, Douglas	*Stroke: A Study of Recovery*	1961	Doubleday and Co., Inc. 501 Franklin Ave New York, New York 11530
Sarno, John E., and Sarno, Martha Taylor	*Stroke — The Condition and the Patient*	1969	McGraw-Hill Book Co. 1221 Ave of the Americas New York, New York 10036
*Smith, Genevieve Waples	*Care of the Patient with a Stroke: A Handbook for the Patient's Family and the Nurse*	1967	Springer Publ Co., Inc. 200 Park Ave. SO. New York, New York 10003
Taylor, Martha L.	*Understanding Aphasia: A Guide for Family and Friends*	1958	Institute of Physical Medicine and Rehabilitation. NYU — Bellevue 400 E. 34th Street New York, New York
Taylor, Martha L., and Marks, Morton M.	*Aphasia Rehabilitation Manual and Therapy Kit (2nd ed.)*		McGraw-Hill Book Co. 1221 Ave of the Americas New York, New York 10036
*Van Rosen, Robert E.	*Comeback: The Story of My Stroke*	1963	Bobbs-Merrill Co., Inc. 4 W. 58th Street New York, New York 10019
*Wint, Guy	*The Third Killer: Meditations on a Stroke*	1967	Abelard-Schuman, Ltd. 257 Park Ave, So. New York, New York 10010
*Wulf, Helen Harlan	*Aphasia, My World Alone*	1973	Wayne State University Press, Detroit, Michigan

*Indicates a self-account or spouse-account.

AUTHOR INDEX

SUBJECT INDEX

M

N

O

P

Q

R

S

T

V

W